An Introduction to the Use of Anticancer Drugs

Commissioning Editor: Heidi Harrison
Development Editor: Catherine Jackson
Project Manager: Joannah Duncan
Designer: Andy Chapman
Illustration Manager: Bruce Hogarth
Illustrator: David Gardner

An Introduction to the Use of Anticancer Drugs

Imran Rafi BSc MBBS MRCPI MRCGP MSc PhD

Principal in General Practice and Senior Lecturer in Primary Care Education
St George's, University of London

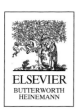

ELSEVIER
BUTTERWORTH
HEINEMANN

Edinburgh • London • New York • Philadelphia • St Louis • Sydney • Toronto 2006

BUTTERWORTH
HEINEMANN

© 2006, Elsevier Limited. All rights reserved.

No part of this publication may be reproduced, stored in a retrieval system, or transmitted in any form or by any means, electronic, mechanical, photocopying, recording or otherwise, without the prior permission of the Publishers. Permissions may be sought directly from Elsevier's Health Sciences Rights Department, 1600 John F. Kennedy Boulevard, Suite 1800, Philadelphia, PA 19103-2899, USA: phone: (+1) 215 239 3804; fax: (+1) 215 239 3805; or, e-mail: *healthpermissions@elsevier.com*. You may also complete your request on-line via the Elsevier homepage (http://www.elsevier.com), by selecting 'Support and contact' and then 'Copyright and Permission'.

First published 2006

ISBN 0 7506 8830 0

British Library Cataloguing in Publication Data
A catalogue record for this book is available from the British Library

Library of Congress Cataloging in Publication Data
A catalog record for this book is available from the Library of Congress

---

Notice

Knowledge and best practice in this field are constantly changing. As new research and experience broaden our knowledge, changes in practice, treatment and drug therapy may become necessary or appropriate. Readers are advised to check the most current information provided (i) on procedures featured or (ii) by the manufacturer of each product to be administered, to verify the recommended dose or formula, the method and duration of administration, and contraindications. It is the responsibility of the practitioner, relying on their own experience and knowledge of the patient, to make diagnoses, to determine dosages and the best treatment for each individual patient, and to take all appropriate safety precautions. To the fullest extent of the law, neither the publisher nor the authors assumes any liability for any injury and/or damage.

The Publisher

Working together to grow
libraries in developing countries

www.elsevier.com | www.bookaid.org | www.sabre.org

ELSEVIER   BOOK AID
International   Sabre Foundation

The
Publisher's
policy is to use
**paper manufactured
from sustainable forests**

Printed in China

ACKNOWLEDGEMENTS

I would like to thank Janine Mansi, Herbie Newell and Fenella Willis for their helpful comments on the manuscript. I would also like to thank my family for remaining ever supportive.

CONTENTS

PREFACE

The aim of this book is to provide an introduction to the principles of drug treatment in cancer medicine. Developments in the understanding of tumour biology, molecular biology and genetics together with the greater understanding of the pharmacology of drugs have combined to open up the field of medical oncology to rapid advances in the treatment of cancers. The range of drugs that are available is wide and one of the primary aims in drug development is to increase the therapeutic window so that drug toxicity is minimised and tolerable. Drug development of oral formulations of anticancer drugs and the use of drugs that could be given in the day patient setting means that healthcare professionals such as General Practitioners who historically might not have been involved in the drug treatment of the cancer patient are now going to need to have a greater understanding of the principles of use of anticancer drugs.

The aim is to give principles of treatment for some of the more common solid tumours rather than the haematological malignancies. The book is intended for

- Medical students
- Doctors in all medical specialties
- General Practitioners
- Pharmacists
- Nurses

Drug doses have largely been omitted as this is not a formulary.

ABBREVIATIONS

ACTH	Adrenocorticotrophic hormone	EMEA	European Agency for Evaluation of Medicinal Products
ADH	Antidiuretic hormone		
AFP	α-fetoprotein	EORTC	European Organisation of Research and Treatment of Cancer
AJCC	American Joint Committee on Cancer		
ALT	Alanine transaminase	ER	Oestrogen receptor
ANC	Absolute neutrophil count	5-FU	5-Fluorouracil
		FBC	Full blood count
AP	Alkaline phosphatase	FDA	Food and Drug Administration
AST	Aspartate transaminases		
AUC	Area under the plasma concentration versus time curve	FIGO	Fédération Internationale de Gynécologie ét d'Obstétrique
		FNA	Fine needle aspiration
BCC	Basal cell carcinoma	G-CSF	Granulocyte colony stimulating factor
BCG	Bacille Calmette–Guérin		
ß-HCG	ß-human chorionic gonadotrophin	GFR	Glomerular filtration rate
		GM-CSF	Granulocyte–macrophage colony stimulating factors
CA-125	Cancer antigen 125		
CEA	Carcinoembryonic antigen	GI	Gastrointestinal
Cr	Creatinine	GMS	General medical services
COG	Clinical Outcomes Group	GTD	Gestational trophoblastic disease
CML	Chronic myeloid leukaemia		
COREC	Central Office for Research Ethics Committees	Hb	Haemoglobin
		HCC	Hepatocellular cancer
CSM	The Committee on Safety of Medicines	hCG	Human chorionic gonadotrophin
CT	Computed tomography	HER	Human epidermal growth factor receptor
CTC	Common Toxicity Criteria		
D&C	Dilatation and curettage	HRQL	Health-related quality of life
DHD	Dihydropyrimidine dehydrogenase	HRT	Hormone replacement therapy
DNA	Deoxyribonuclic acid	ICON	The International Collaborative Ovarian Neoplasm Group
DPD	Dihydropyrimidine dehydrogenase		
DVT	Deep vein thrombosis	IFN	Interferon
EC	European Community	IL	Interleukin
EDTA	Ethylenediaminetetra-acetic acid	INR	International normalised ratio
EGFR	Epidermal growth factor receptor	i.m	Intramuscular
		i.p	Intrapertitoneal
EGFR-TK	Epidermal growth factor receptor-tyrosine kinase	i.v.	Intravenous
		IVU	Intravenous urogram

LDH	Lactate dehydrogenase	PET	Positron emission
LFT	Liver function test		tomography
LH	Luteinising hormone	PLDH	Pegylated liposomal
LHRH	Luteinising hormone-releasing		doxorubicin hydrochloride
	hormone	p.o.	per oral
LREC	Local Research Ethics	PS	Performance status
	Committee	PSA	Prostate-specific antigen
MUGA	Multiple gated acquisition	RT	Radiotherapy
	(scan)	RECIST	Response Evaluation Criteria
NSAIDs	Non-steroidal anti-		in Solid Tumours (the
	inflammatory drugs		published rules that define
MDR	Multidrug resistance		the response of cancers to
mg	Milligrams		treatment)
µg/mL	Microgram per millilitre	s.c.	Subcutaneous
mRNA	Messenger ribonucleic acid	SCC	Squamous cell carcinoma
MHRA	Medicines and Healthcare	SCLC	Small cell lung cancer
	Products Regulatory Agency	SERM	Selective oestrogen receptor
MRC	Medical Research Council		modulators
MREC	Multiple Research Ethics	SHA	Strategic Health Authority
	Committee	SIADH	Syndrome of inappropriate
MRI	Magnetic resonance imaging		antidiuretic hormone
MTD	Maximum tolerated dose	SPMS	Specialist primary medical
MTX	Methotrexate		services
NCI	National Cancer Institute	$t_{1/2}$	Half-life
NCRI	The National Cancer	TGF	Tumour growth factor
	Research Institute	TNM	Tumour, node, metastasis
NCRNCC	The National Cancer		(staging system for cancer)
	Research Network	TS	Thymidylate synthase
	Coordinating Centre	U&E	Urea and electrolytes
NHS	National Health Service	UKCCCR	The United Kingdom
NICE	National Institute for Clinical		Co-ordinating Committee on
	Excellence		Cancer Research
NSCLC	Non-small-cell lung cancer	VEGF	Vascular endothelial growth
NTRAC	National Translational Cancer		factor
	Research Network	WCC	White cell count
PCT	Primary care trust	WHO	World Health Organization

GLOSSARY

OF TERMS IN RELATION TO CANCER CHEMOTHERAPY

Adjuvant therapy Chemotherapy or hormonal drugs given after surgery and/or radiotherapy to eradicate micrometastatic disease.

Area under the curve This area under a plot of plasma drug concentration against time after drug administration. The area can be determined by the trapezoidal rule. It is used particularly in estimating the total drug clearance and in estimating the bioavailability of the drug.

Bioavailability The percentage of a dose of an oral drug that enters the systemic circulation after administration of a given dose compared with an intravenous administration of drug.

Dose This is the quantity of drug administered and may be an absolute dose or a relative dose such as mg/m².

Half-life The time it takes for the concentration or the amount of drug to be reduced to one-half of a given dose administered. The half-life is dependent on which fluid or tissue the drug is being distributed in, e.g. plasma half-life. The pharmacokinetics of the drug determines the half-life. For example a drug that is slowly metabolised tends to circulate longer.

Growth factors Colony stimulating factors that help stimulate bone marrow production after treatment with chemotherapy or radiotherapy.

Neoadjuvant Chemotherapeutic or hormonal drugs given before surgery and/or radiotherapy to reduce tumour bulk.

Pharmacodynamics The study of how drugs affect the body.

Pharmacogenetics The relationship between the pharmacokinetics and pharmacodynamics of a drug. It is dependent on the genetic profile and attributes of drug handling.

Pharmacokinetics The study of drug absorption, distribution, metabolism and clearance of a drug.

Prodrug A chemical that, in normal circumstances, does not produce a pharmacological effect but when administered is transformed into an active drug in the body.

Remission Complete or partial response to the symptoms or signs of cancer.

Renal clearance The volume of plasma or blood that is cleared of a substance by renal mechanisms alone in a unit of time. This can be dependent on renal function, the age of the patient, the weight, cardiovascular factors and gender.

Salvage treatment The use of another form of treatment after failure of the primary treatment.

OF CHEMOTHERAPY REGIMENS

ABVD – Doxorubicin, bleomycin, vinblastine, dacarbazine

ABCM – Adriamycin® (doxorubicin), BCNU, cyclophosphamide and melphalan

AC – Adriamycin® (doxorubicin) and cyclophosphamide

ACE – Adriamycin® (doxorubicin), cyclophosphamide and etoposide

BEACOPP – Bleomycin, etoposide, doxorubicin, cyclophosphamide, vincristine, procarbazine and prednisolone

BEP – Bleomycin, etoposide and cisplatin

CAP – Cyclophosphamide, doxorubicin and cisplatin

CEB – Carboplatin, etoposide and bleomycin

ChlVPP – Chlorambucil, vinblastine, procarbazine and prednisolone

CHOP – Cyclophosphamide, vincristine, doxorubicin and prednisolone

CMF – Cyclophosphamide, methotrexate and 5-fluorouracil

CVAMP – Cyclophosphamide, vincristine, Adriamycin® (doxorubicin) and methylprednisolone

CVP – Cyclophosphamide, vincristine and prednisolone

EC – Epirubicin and cyclophosphamide

ECF – Epirubicin, cisplatin and 5-fluorouracil

ELF – Etoposide, folinic acid (leucovorin), and 5-fluorouracil

EMACO – Etoposide, actinomycin-D, methotrexate, vincristine and cyclophosphamide

FAMTX – 5-fluorouracil, doxorubicin and high-dose methotrexate.

FAC – Fluorouracil with Adriamycin® (doxorubicin) and cyclophosphamide

FEC – Fluorouracil, epirubicin and cyclophosphamide

Fluorouracil regimens (in colorectal cancers):

- Mayo Clinic regimen: The bolus 5-fluorouracil and folinic acid regimen of 5-fluorouracil 425 mg/m^2/day i.v. days 1–5 and leucovorin 20 mg/m^2/day i.v. days 1–5 both repeated every 4–5 weeks for 6 months

- De Gramont regimen: Leucovorin 200 mg/m^2 as a 2-hour infusion days 1 and 2. 5-Fluorouracil 400 mg/m^2 i.v. then 5-fluorouracil 600 mg/m^2 continuous infusion over 22 hours days 1 and 2. Repeated every 14 days

- Lokich regimen: 5-Fluorouracil 300 mg/m^2/day by continuous i.v. infusion until toxicity or disease progression

GC – Gemcitabine and cisplatin

ICE – Ifosfamide, carboplatin and etoposide

MIC – Mitomycin, ifosfamide and cisplatin

MOPP – Nitrogen mustard, vincristine, procarbazine and prednisolone

MP – Melphalan and prednisolone

MVAC – Methotrexate, vinblastine, Adriamycin® (doxorubicin) and cisplatin

MVP – Mitomycin, vindesine or vinblastine and cisplatin

PABIOE – Prednisolone, Adriamycin® (doxorubicin), bleomycin, vincristine (Oncovin®) and etoposide

PCV – Procarbazine, CCNU and vincristine

PmitCEBO – Prednisolone, mitoxantrone, cyclophosphamide, etoposide, bleomycin and vincristine

VAPEC-B – Vincristine, Adriamycin® (doxorubicin), prednisolone, etoposide, cyclophosphamide and bleomycin

VAD – Vincristine, Adriamycin® (doxorubicin) and dexamethasone

CHAPTER 1

Introduction to anticancer drugs

INTRODUCTION: PRINCIPLES

Anticancer drugs comprise one of the three principal modalities of treatment offered to a patient with a malignancy, the other two being surgery and radiotherapy. Surgery is the main initial treatment for a number of malignancies, including breast cancer, colorectal cancer, head and neck cancers, skin cancers and testicular cancers. Adjuvant surgery can be achieved by the removal of apparently normal tissue surrounding the tumour to prevent local recurrence.

Radiotherapy has developed through an understanding of radiobiology and technical advances. It is used for three primary purposes. First, the radical treatment of malignancy with curative intent, such as in the treatment of Hodgkin's disease. Second, in adjuvant therapy, as in breast cancer. And third, in the palliative treatment of malignancy to reduce symptoms and help pain control, such as in bone metastases.

The third treatment modality – chemotherapy – now encompasses a broad range of agents that range from hormonal therapy to the use of therapy targeting the molecular basis of cancer. Adjuvant drug therapy has been used to prevent micrometastatic spread, as in the treatment of breast and colorectal cancer. Cancers have now become curable through drug treatment. Combination drug treatment can cure cancers, as in the case of childhood cancers and rare adult tumours. The use of combination chemotherapy before surgery with postoperative radiotherapy in primary osteosarcoma illustrates the importance of a multidisciplinary approach to the treatment of cancer. The involvement of the medical and clinical oncologist, surgical oncologist, radiologists and palliative care teams working together at the time of diagnosis as part of a multidisciplinary team will enable treatment to be matched to the needs of the patient.

ENHANCING DRUG TREATMENT

Only a small number of all cancers are curable with available therapies. The two main limitations faced when treating malignancy are the lack of selectivity of antitumour agents and the inherent resistance of tumour cells. Improved selectivity with new molecularly-targeted anticancer agents aims to reduce host toxicity by selective tumour cell kill. Conversely, advances in reducing host toxicity include the development of haematopoietic growth factors such as colony-stimulating factors, which enable host 'rescue' from bone marrow suppressive drugs. In turn, improved haematopoietic support allows dose intensification to be explored, although it has not been proved beyond doubt that dose intensification leads to improved survival. A further way to enhance drug action is biochemical modulation, which relies on the understanding and manipulation of the key metabolic processes involved in drug action. In certain malignancies, such as colon cancer, biochemical modulation has been used to achieve a greater response rate.

DRUG RESISTANCE

Drug resistance remains a common clinical problem that dictates overall response to chemotherapy. Inherent resistance is the failure of a tumour to respond to the first chemotherapy given, e.g. the majority of non-small-cell lung cancers. In acquired resistance, tumours respond initially but then become refractory to further therapy, e.g. small cell lung cancer. Cellular resistance is dictated by a multitude of factors but two critical parameters are inadequate drug concentrations either at the site of action, and hence levels of target interaction, and an impaired apoptotic response in the tumour cell. Factors that can reduce the availability of a drug at the molecular target include reduced cellular uptake of drug, drug efflux pumps such as P-glycoprotein, which is sited on the cell membrane and which acts to pump out drug from the cell or intracellular detoxification, e.g. by glutathione, which can act to prevent DNA damage. Activation of repair mechanisms, as in the case of DNA repair enzymes, can antagonise the effect of anticancer drugs. When malignant cells express genes, which suppress apoptosis, or programmed cell death, then these cells may not undergo drug-induced apoptosis. For example, BCL-2 expression, initially identified as a translocated gene product in follicular lymphoma, has been shown to delay the onset of apoptosis induced by almost all classes of cytotoxic drugs. Other more specific resistance mechanisms depend on the pharmacological properties of the drug being administered. Tumour cell kinetics help determine at what point anticancer drugs are likely to have an impact to prevent cellular proliferation. The pharmacokinetics of the drug are clearly important in determining whether there are sites where drug concentrations may be suboptimal for an antitumour effect.

PHARMACOKINETICS AND PHARMACODYNAMICS

With respect to systemic determinants of drug action, it is important, when administering any drug, to understand the pharmacokinetics and pharmacodynamics of the agent. Pharmacokinetics involves drug absorption, metabolism and elimination. An understanding of the pharmacokinetics of the drug can allow optimisation of effective drug delivery and hence therapy.

Pharmacodynamics concerns studies of the end-organ effects of the drug and includes both toxicity and the therapeutic actions of the drug. The dose, dose rate and schedule of drug administration all have a large influence on drug efficacy in oncology. A measure of drug exposure that is often used is the area under the plasma concentration versus time curve (AUC). Relationships between pharmacokinetics (e.g. AUC) and pharmacodynamics (e.g. percentage change in platelet count parameters) have been described (e.g. for carboplatin). These relationships can be used prospectively to minimise toxicity and maximise activity.

A drug can produce a pharmacological action in four main ways (Turner et al 1986):

1. Interaction with specific receptors, as exemplified by the action of the hormonal drugs, which exert an agonist effect on specific receptors and thus result in a biological response. Partial agonists and competitive antagonists work to reduce the effect of the drug on its receptor reducing the efficacy of the drug.
2. Pharmacodynamically by inhibiting certain enzymes. An example of this is methotrexate, a drug that works to compete with dihydrofolate for the intracellular enzyme dihydrofolate reductase.
3. By intracellular activation and reaction with macromolecules, such as the action of the platinum compounds, which form DNA adducts that bind to DNA and prevent replication.
4. By a direct physical action, such as the use of charcoal in the treatment of poisoning.

The scheduling of drugs depends on the pharmacology of the drug being administered. The aim is to allow recovery from the effects of treatment while maximising an antiproliferative effect on tumour cells. This relies on knowledge of how the drug acts and tumour cell growth and the cell cycle.

RELATIONSHIP BETWEEN CHEMOTHERAPY AND TUMOUR GROWTH

A tumour develops from a cancer cell that has arisen from a cell that has undergone a malignant transformation. For a cell to thrive it requires a good blood supply, oxygen and nutrition. At a critical mass the rate of growth reduces because of cellular hypoxia due to poor blood supply; the larger the tumour becomes, the slower the rate of growth. Thus tumours with proliferating cells are most likely to respond to chemotherapy and those tumours with slowly dividing cells are least likely to respond to chemotherapy.

The Goldie–Colman model suggests that there is tumour heterogeneity due to the development of spontaneous cellular mutations. Thus those cells most susceptible to chemotherapy are those where there is a low tumour bulk and combinations of drugs are used to overcome tumour resistance. Repeated treatments will decrease the tumour size and hence the need to schedule a drug whether it be given orally, i.v. bolus or as an i.v. infusion. One principle of adjuvant therapy after surgery or radiotherapy is that by reducing tumour bulk, the residual tumour has faster growing cells and hence more likely to respond to chemotherapy.

THE MALIGNANT CELLS AND MOLECULAR TARGETS

New drugs commonly are now arising from rational drug design based on a better understanding of the molecular biology and genetics of cancer.

The normal balance between cell proliferation and growth and cell death is lost in cancer, and the normal cell relies on signals that maintain the regulatory balance. The multistep theory of carcinogenesis suggests that a number of genetic mutations in the DNA of somatic cells are necessary before a clinically-detectable cancer develops. The key genes that are involved in cancer development are oncogenes and tumour suppressor genes.

Proto-oncogenes are genes that promote normal cell growth and division. The protein products of proto-oncogenes are the signals that are necessary for cell growth. Mutation of proto-oncogenes to oncogenes results in uncontrolled cell growth and division (Fig. 1.1). Mutation of a gene may occur through chromosomal changes, point mutations and gene amplification and oncogenes normally act as a dominant phenotype. An example of an oncogene is the erb B2, or HER2/neu, oncogene, which is a growth factor found in some breast, ovarian and lung cancers.

The role of tumour suppressor cells is normally to negatively regulate cell growth and division. An example of an important tumour suppressor gene is the p53 gene. It can limit cell proliferation by affecting the cell cycle or activating apoptosis. Mutations in the wild-type p53 lead to cell proliferation, which can result in the accumulation of defective cells with damaged DNA leading to tumour formation. Additional examples of the tumour suppressor

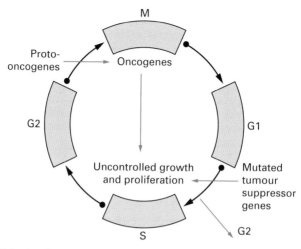

Fig. 1.1 Cell cycle and tumour growth.

gene are the BRCA1 gene (which is associated with familial breast and ovarian cancer), BRCA2 (also involved in hereditary breast cancer) and the APC gene (involved with familial adenomatous polyposis of the colon).

THE CELL CYCLE AND TUMOUR GROWTH

Normal control of cell division depends on the cell cycle:

- GAP1 (G1), when cells prepare for DNA replication
- synthesis of DNA (S)
- GAP2 (G2), when RNA and proteins are produced
- mitosis (M), when cell division occurs.

There is also a resting phase (G0) from which cells can either re-enter the cell cycle or terminally differentiate. Mutations in proto-oncogenes, tumour suppressor genes or DNA repair genes can lead to uncontrolled cell growth.

Once cell cycle control is lost, cells may proliferate with undifferentiated potential for growth. The development of a tumour from the initial transformed cells also relies on the balance between the factors that stimulate angiogenesis, the production of new blood vessels to sustain the tumour and antiangiogenic factors that counteract this process. Tumour invasion occurs when the normal architecture between cells – the extracellular matrix – is lost with the subsequent development of metastasis through local invasion into lymphatic and vascular structures.

APOPTOSIS OR PROGRAMMED CELL DEATH

Apoptosis is the process of programmed cell death. Mutations loss of normal control mechanisms for apoptosis lead to increased cell survival in cancer. The protein product of p53 can influence apoptosis, the cell cycle and DNA repair processes. Cytotoxic chemotherapy and hormonal therapy attempts to induce apoptosis in tumour cells by causing cellular damage or block growth stimulation by hormones and this may be dependent on p53 mechanisms. The corollary of this is that resistance to drug action may occur if there are mutations in apoptotic pathways. For example, mutations in p53 may be associated with drug resistance particularly in breast and ovarian cancer. Chemotherapy agents that do not cause DNA damage, such as the taxanes, may trigger apoptosis through p53-independent pathways.

In the future it may be that anticancer therapy may be dictated by the patient's genetic profile and the molecular profile of the cancer.

MOLECULAR TARGETS AND CHEMOTHERAPY

The principles of pharmacogenomics (how the individual's genetic inheritance affects the body's response to drugs) and pharmacogenetics (the study of the hereditary basis for differences in populations' response to a drug) may be used to identify patients who are at an increased risk for toxicity or who may be sensitive to cytotoxic therapies (Chabner 2002).

An individual patient-tailored form of treatment may be possible by identifying polymorphisms or variations in the genome and matching these to the pharmacokinetics and pharmacodynamics of anticancer agents. For example, it is known that some patients suffer from severe toxicity associated with the antimetabolite 5-Fluorouracil (5-FU). This is because they are deficient in dihydropyrimidine dehydrogenase (DPD) activity, which is a key enzyme and rate-limiting step in the degradation pathway of 5-FU. By identifying these patients through genetic molecular analysis it would be possible to identify those who might be susceptible to severe toxicity.

CLASSIFICATION OF CYTOTOXIC DRUGS

Cytotoxic drugs can be classified according to their mechanisms of action:

- The alkylating agents act by formation of DNA adducts by alkylation of the base residues in nucleic acid, e.g. cyclophosphamide and melphalan. They can be further subdivided into groups depending on their chemical structures, e.g. nitrogen mustards, nitrosureas.
- The platinum agents, e.g. cisplatin and carboplatin, which form DNA adducts leading to apoptotic cell death.

- The antitumour antibiotics include the anthracyclines (e.g. doxorubicin) and non-anthracyclines (bleomycin). Anthracyclines bind to DNA and can cause inhibition of topoisomerase II function, a nuclear enzyme involved in DNA processing.
- The epipodophylotoxins, i.e. etoposide, also cause DNA strand breaks by forming complexes with topoisomerase II.
- The tubulin binders, which either inhibit (e.g. vinca alkaloids) or stabilise (e.g. taxanes) microtubule formation and tubulin polymerisation. Tubulin is an important structural protein in mitosis.
- The antimetabolites, which interfere with RNA and DNA synthesis by either acting as substrates for or inhibiting enzymes involved in nucleotide biosynthesis.
- Miscellaneous groups, which include camptothecin analogues such as irinotecan, which inhibit the DNA top-isomerase I enzyme, and the retinoids are an example of a differentiation agent that prevents the cell from entering the cell cycle and have been used in the treatment of leukaemia (e.g. all-*trans*-retinoic acid).

HORMONAL AGENTS

The hormonal manipulation of cancer by endocrine therapy of cancer is used for a range of cancers including prostate and breast cancer. There is a wide range of common endocrine therapy used in treating cancer or used for palliation:

- steroids
- aromatase inhibitors
- antiandrogens
- luteinising hormone-releasing hormone (LHRH) analogues
- oestrogen-receptor antagonists
- progestogens
- somatostatin analogues.

Hormonal therapy may act as an agonist or antagonist to affect the hormone-sensitive tumour. Breast, prostate, renal, uterine and thyroid cancers are sensitive to hormonal manipulation. For example, the actions of oestrogens in breast cancer and testosterone in prostate cancer can adversely affect outcome, and the use of hormonal agents that counter the effects of these hormones are used as part of treatment. Endocrine therapy using adrenal corticosteroids is used in the treatment of a number of tumours, especially in the haematological malignancies. Endocrine therapy can also be used as an aid for palliating symptoms, e.g. progestins as appetite stimulants. Chapter 3 describes how endocrine therapy works at a cellular level and the range of hormonal agents that are used in the treatment of cancers.

BIOLOGICAL THERAPIES AND IMMUNOTHERAPY

Immunotherapy, or biological response modifier therapy, uses knowledge about the immune system as either an anticancer therapy or in an attempt to lessen side effects of chemotherapy and radiotherapy treatments. The types of cell used in immunotherapy programmes include lymphocytes (including B cells), T cells and natural killer cells:

- B cells develop into plasma cells that produce antibodies to form antibody–antigen complexes.
- T lymphocytes can be divided into cytotoxic T cells and helper T cells, both of which are able to produce proteins called cytokines. Cytokines have an immunomodulating effect on the immune system and are subdivided into colony stimulating factors, interferons, interleukins and lymphokines.
- Natural killer cells act quickly in the presence of antigens to produce cytokines to lead to lysis of cells. Phagocytosis is the process whereby circulating monocytes and tissue macrophages engulf and digest microscopic organisms.

Biological therapies are a new modality in the treatment of cancer. They are used as sole agents or in combination treatment, either as an anticancer agent or as an immunomodulator to aid recovery from myelosuppressive treatment. Biological response modifiers can be classified as:

- Interferons (IFNs): these are naturally occurring cytokines and can be subdivided into three types of natural IFNs: alpha (α), beta (β) and gamma (γ). They have shown activity in cancer treatment and also in the treatment of autoimmune disease, and are naturally produced in response to viral infections. The range of use of interferon-α, for example, varies from the treatment of malignant melanoma and hairy cell leukaemia to the treatment of chronic hepatitis B infections. Interferons have also been used as part of combination therapy with cytotoxic agents.
- Interleukins (ILs): these naturally occurring cytokines can act as leucocyte mediators, stimulating the immune system. Interleukin-2 (IL-2) is used in the treatment of metastatic renal cell carcinoma and metastatic melanoma.
- Colony stimulating factors: these are growth factors acting on the haematopoietic system to stimulate bone marrow stem cells to divide. Erythropoietin, granulocyte colony stimulating factors (G-CSF) and granulocyte–macrophage colony stimulating factors (GM-CSF) are examples of colony stimulating factors. The former stimulates red cell production and the latter two stimulate white cell production. Their use ranges across a range of tumour types, particularly when severe myelosuppression occurs as a result of treatment and leads to febrile neutropenia, or in randomised trials, particularly in the use of high-dose chemotherapy.
- Monoclonal antibodies: made by fusing an antibody-producing B cell to a fast-growing cell, e.g. a cancerous myeloma cell. The resulting hybrid cell,

or hybridoma, multiplies rapidly. This in turn produces a large quantity of a clonal antibody. Herceptin® (trastuzumab) is an example of an monoclonal antibody used to treat metastatic breast cancer in patients with tumours that produce excess amounts of a protein called HER2 and work, by blocking HER2 recptors.

- Cancer vaccines: cancer vaccines are produced from cellular cancer related-proteins or genes are used to stimulate the immune system. Trials are underway in malignant melanoma, renal cell cancers as well as colon, breast and prostate cancers. A range of different types of vaccine is being produced and undergoing clinical trials including the use of allogenic and autologous vaccines, dendritic and anti-idiotype vaccines.

- Gene therapy: using DNA and clonal techniques it is possible to manipulate cells to introduce new genetic code to produce specific proteins. The vehicles to reintroduce altered genetic material into the body include the use of liposomes and viruses. There may be many reasons to do this. For example, to repair defective tumour suppressor genes, such as p53, or the use of antisense oligonucleotides, which are pieces of genetic material introduced to block gene expression. An example is the case of the bcl-2 gene expressed in follicular lymphoma where its action is to block apoptosis. Antisense oligonucleotides blocking gene transcription to bcl-2 is a new treatment considered for lymphoma and are undergoing clinical studies although these have yet to show any benefit.

- Non-specific immunomodulating agents: these agents stimulate or modulate the immune system. The aim is to stimulate target immune system cells and cause lead to an increased production of cytokines and immunoglobulin. An example of such agents includes bacille Calmette–Guérin (BCG). BCG is used in the treatment of superficial bladder cancer, usually after surgery where it leads to an inflammatory reaction.

- Angiogenesis inhibitors and the inhibitors of matrix metalloproteinase: angiogenesis depends on growth factors that stimulate the production of new blood vessels. Working against this are factors that inhibit this process. New antiangiogenic factors are undergoing trials at the moment, as are old established drugs that have been shown to have antiangiogenic properties, such as thalidomide. Inhibitors of the protein matrix metalloproteinase, which break down extra cellular matrix, are being evaluated in clinical trials.

PRINCIPLES OF COMBINATION CHEMOTHERAPY

There are several reasons why there is a need to combine different drugs to optimise the chance of inducing apoptosis or death of the cancer cell. If a drug is found to be active against a particular tumour, then pre-clinical in vitro and in vivo studies can help determine if combinations of drugs are more active. Furthermore, combinations of drugs may act synergistically and through different mechanisms of action. Combination of drugs that have different toxicities allows the administration of drugs at near top doses. Similarly, drugs can be beneficially combined if they have different resistance profiles and different toxicity profiles.

WHEN TO GIVE CHEMOTHERAPY

Adjuvant chemotherapy is used when there is no residual disease after removal of the primary tumour and usually involves the systemic administration of chemotherapy drugs. This differs from neoadjuvant chemotherapy, which is the use of chemotherapy before removal of local disease. Adjuvant therapy has been established in the treatment of breast cancer, lung cancer, colorectal cancer, osteosarcoma, ovarian cancer, testicular cancer, bladder cancer and the treatment of melanoma. Examples of when neoadjuvant therapy is given is in the treatment of cervical cancer using chemotherapy to debulk the tumour before radical surgery or in breast cancer to downstage large tumours to facilitate conservative surgery as opposed to mastectomy.

Toxicities associated with adjuvant therapy are an important consideration when selecting patients who might benefit from treatment. These toxicities range from the short-term side effects such as gastrointestinal (GI) symptoms to long-term ones such as the risk of secondary malignancies. An example of a late complication is the need to monitor for breast cancer after original treatment for Hodgkin's lymphoma.

Quality of life issues are an important consideration in making a decision about the need to start adjuvant chemotherapy. The potential advantages of adjuvant therapy include the eradication of microscopic metastatic disease, although postoperative recovery may delay the timing of therapy.

Palliative chemotherapy is used to maintain quality of life and control symptoms. Stable disease over a 6-month period is important in terms of symptom palliation. However, there should be acceptable toxicity to give effective control of disease progression. Patients also may be quite variable in their emotional response to the side effects of treatment. For example, a woman receiving Taxol® chemotherapy might be distraught about the effects of neurotoxicity leading to a peripheral neuropathy because she is unable to do fine artwork; her alopecia may be less of a problem.

How chemotherapy is administered is also important. Patients needing intravenous lines, including Hickman lines, can find the process of chemotherapy administration difficult, time-consuming and restrictive. Development of oral formulations of drugs that have a similar efficacy of action to intravenous chemotherapy can therefore improve the quality of the life of a cancer patient.

Few studies have looked at the benefit of home-based chemotherapy and economics, ease of administration, patient factors and nursing time are all important facets of determining how feasible this might be. Furthermore there are patient education and training aspects of care.

CLINICAL TRIALS AND CANCER NETWORKS IN THE UK

KEY DEVELOPMENTS IN THE ORGANISATION OF CANCER CARE IN THE UK

An expert advisory group was established to prepare a policy framework for commissioning cancer services in 1995. The guiding principles were driven by the need to deliver quality care; to detect early cancers; to better communicate between patients and professionals; to involve primary care in primary prevention, early screening, diagnosis and palliative care; and to set up cancer registers, particularly to monitor outcomes. The **Calman/Hine report** (Calman & Hine 1995) recommended the setting-up of cancer networks, which would organise cancer services that would cover care from primary care through to cancer centres. There would be three levels of care: (i) primary care; (ii) cancer units, usually in district general hospitals; and (iii) designated cancer centres, which would be serving regional areas with diagnostic and therapeutic expertise. The theme was to harness the advantages of multidisciplinary teams to achieve better treatment of cancers.

In particular, it was recommended that the administration of chemotherapy should be done in a cancer unit only if there were facilities, standards and treatment protocols delivered by multidisciplinary teams. A lead clinician would coordinate the range of services provided within a cancer unit. The cancer centre would serve a regional area providing a specialist range of services and management of a wide spectrum of cancer treatment, including complex cancer intensive surgery, radiotherapy and the more inpatient chemotherapy and diagnostic techniques. To aid primary care management of cancers it was recommended that local guidelines be developed to ensure good communication between primary and secondary care, particularly after discharge of the patient from the cancer unit or centre. GPs can refer patients with suspected cancers to be seen within 2 weeks of the referral being made. The aim of all these changes was to set up a network system to bring together all cancer services in a regional area. Throughout the UK there are now 34 cancer networks.

The initial problem was implementing the findings of the report. There were no extra resources and no central organising body that would help to implement the changes recommended. Each individual region was expected to draw up proposals relevant to local needs. National guidance was provided by the Clinical Outcomes Group (COG), which helped to produce guidance by multidisciplinary experts on the management of tumour specific cancers.

From 1997, cancer services and delivery of treatment were given a higher priority and more central coordination of cancer services than before. This led to the **NHS Cancer Plan** (2000). The aim of the NHS Cancer Plan was to help deliver a strategy to tackle cancer, prevention, screening, diagnosis, treatment, and research and development. It recognised the need to provide the infrastructure in terms of staff and equipment. It stipulated the need to target smoking, reduce waiting times for treatment and to invest in palliative care. One of its primary aims was to eradicate inequalities in the care of patients with cancer throughout the UK. The cancer networks were responsible for delivering the objectives.

The **National Cancer Research Institute** (NCRI) was formed in 2001 as a partnership between the government and the research charities and the private sector. There were three main aims of the NCRI: (i) to take a strategic overview of cancer research in the UK; (ii) to identify gaps in cancer research; and (iii) to facilitate collaboration between the cancer research funding bodies. Members of the NCRI include Cancer Research UK, The Medical Research Council (MRC) and Leukaemia Research Fund. A number of criteria need to be met before an organisation can become an active member of the NCRI. These are: (i) to be a funder of cancer research in the UK; (ii) to have a budget for annual cancer research in the UK in excess of £1 million; and (iii) to have an appropriate, peer-reviewed system for maintaining the scientific quality of funded research.

The **National Cancer Research Network, Coordinating Centre** (NCRN, CC) was set up in 2001 to coordinate the 34 cancer research networks. The initial aim was to double the number of incident cases entering clinical trials and, in the long term, to increase the accrual rate for clinical trials to 10% for incident cases. It operates, under the strategic overview of the NCRI, as a network that matches the NHS cancer service networks in England. One of its roles is to coordinate the running of the NCRI Clinical Studies Groups, which are peer-reviewed groups acting as a resource in the management of specific tumour areas to promote high quality research. A cancer research database has been set up to provide information on research projects funded by the NCRI members.

The aim of the **National Translational Cancer Research Network** (NTRAC), the sister organisation of the NCRI, is to coordinate a national programme of translational cancer research whereby novel anticancer therapeutics and diagnostics are translated form the laboratory to clinical trials as soon as possible.

The **United Kingdom Coordinating Committee on Cancer Research** (UKCCCR) maintains the National Register of Cancer Clinical Trials, which is a register of hundreds of past and present randomised controlled trials in cancer (the register is available online at: www.ctu.mrc.ac.uk/ukcccr/home.asp).

The **Cancer Collaborative Project** was also set up to pilot an improvement model for change in specific areas developed by the Institute of Healthcare Improvement in the USA. In terms of treatment, its aim was to assess delivery of care by assessing the multidisciplinary approach to treatment. It has had some success in improvement of local services.

The remit of the **National Institute of Clinical Excellence** (NICE) is to be an independent organisation providing guidance on aspects of care in

England and Wales as part of the NHS. It appraises new drug treatments and technology through an evidence base. It produces clinical guidelines and guidance on interventional procedures. The full list of currently (2005) published guidance of drugs appraised by NICE in relation to cancer chemotherapy treatment to data is listed below:

- brain: temozolomide
- breast: capectiabine, docetaxel, paclitaxel, trastuzumab, vinorelbine
- colorectal: capecitabine, irinotecan, oxaliplatin, ralitrexed, tefagur
- lung: docetaxel, gemcitabine, paclitaxel, vinorelbine
- haematological: fludarabine, imatinab, riluximab
- ovarian: docetaxel, paclitaxel, DLDH (Caelyx™), topotecan
- pancreatic: gemcitabine.

The research charity **Cancer Research UK** was formed following on from merger of the Cancer Research Campaign and the Imperial Cancer Research Fund in 2002. Its remit is to support research groups through direct grants and support for research institutes. The *British Journal of Cancer* is owned by Cancer Research UK (see Appendix 1).

The purpose of the **UK Clinical Research Collaboration** is to promote clinical trial work in the UK in all therapeutic areas. It will work on the same model used by the cancer research networks and encourage collaboration between primary care trusts, industry and clinicians.

Professor Mike Richards was appointed **National Cancer Director** in 1999. The aim of this appointment by the Department of Health is to take on the national priorities in the delivery of good quality cancer care and treatment. The National Cancer Director is accountable to ministers and was commissioned by the Secretary of State for Health in 2003 to look at the variation of cancer drug prescribing and deviations from NICE recommendations across England, and the reasons why there might be a so-called postcode lottery in the prescribing of drugs (see: www.dh.gov.uk/). The stakeholders involved in this consultation process were the cancer networks, Strategic Health Authorities (SHAs) and the pharmaceutical industry. The remit of the report was to look at reported variations in the usage of 16 cancer drugs appraised by NICE and, using comparator drugs, identify the reasons for variations and decide an action plan to ensure that patients have access to NICE-approved cancer drugs. The key findings were that: (i) overall use of anticancer drugs does increase following positive appraisal from NICE and (ii) there are many reasons for variations in prescribing, the main one being service delivery constraints and variations in clinical practice. Differences in case mix do not account for the variation.

The government's reply to these findings came in a letter from Lord Warner, the Parliamentary Under Secretary of State (Warner 2004). An action plan was proposed to deliver and implement NICE recommendations and guidelines. These included general themes of selecting topics for NICE appraisal that were relevant to NHS priorities, developing further guidance, more effective dissemination of information from NICE that was relevant to professionals and patients, and enhancing feedback and monitoring systems, including the use of electronic prescribing.

PRIMARY CARE TRUSTS AND PRIMARY CARE

A recent House of Commons Select Committee Report by the Science and Technology Group highlighted the problem in delivering resources and funding through the Primary Care Trusts (PCTs) to the cancer networks. At present, there are over 300 PCTs in England and over three-quarters of the NHS budget is held by the PCTs. Cancer care commissioning is done by the commissioners of the PCTs and it is unlikely that recent changes in primary care legislation allowing practice-based commissioning or specialist primary medical services (SPMS) will influence who does commissioning for cancer services in view of the complexity of the treatment of cancer care. The all-party Parliamentary Group on Cancer called for powers for commissioning cancer treatment to be taken away from primary care trusts (PCTs). The report was highlighted at the Britain Against Cancer Conference in 2004. The recommendation was that the extra funding for cancer standing at around £500 million should be handed over to the cancer networks. One of the criticisms was so-called 'postcode lottery' in prescribing of anticancer drugs, with variations in access to anticancer drugs as highlighted by the National Cancer Director. The call was that there should be specialist cancer commissioning.

A recent report evaluated the role and experience of PCT cancer leads (Centre for Research in Primary Care 2004). These lead clinicians had 3 years of funding from the Department of Health and were supported by Macmillan Cancer Relief. Their main role was seen as strategic within the local cancer network. Although there was a focus on palliative care, one of their achievements was to raise awareness of cancer in primary care and work closely with the providers within the network.

The new General Medical Services Contract (2004) for GPs highlights cancer care management. It may make a difference to the care of cancer patients in the community by the setting-up of disease registers and by ensuring that each patient in the community has a review of the cancer care he or she is receiving. The NHS Plan cites the National Primary Care Development Team and the Modernisation Agency (NHS 2001) as bodies that should work with PCTs and GPs to improve the care of patients in terms of looking at capacity and demand and the primary/secondary interface.

EUROPEAN AND US COLLABORATIVE ORGANISATIONS

European Organisation of Research and Treatment of Cancer (EORTC) (www.eortc.be)

This organisation is one of the largest European cancer clinical trials networks. Its activities include the coordination of laboratory and clinical research in Europe. It also undertakes some collaborative work with the US National Cancer Institute and Cancer Research UK.

The US National Cancer Institute (NCI)

The National Cancer Institute (NCI) is the US government's principal agency for cancer research and training. The National Cancer Act of 1971 created the National Cancer Program and the National Cancer Institute coordinates the National Cancer Program. This involves supporting research, education, training and public information in cancer. The range is wide and covers prevention, diagnosis and treatment of cancer. It supports a network of cancer centres across the USA, like the UK model.

References

Calman K, Hine D 1995 A policy framework for commissioning cancer services: a report by the expert advisory group on cancer to the chief medical officers of England and Wales. Department of Health, London

Centre for Research in Primary Care 2004 Early days yet. The primary care cancer lead clinician (PCCL) initiative. Executive summary. University of Leeds, Leeds

Chabner BA 2002 Cytotoxic agents in the era of molecular targets and genomics. The Oncologist 7(Suppl 3):34–41

Lord Warner 2004 Implementation of NICE guidance. Department of Health, London

NHS 2000 The NHS Cancer Plan. 2000 Online. Available at: www.publications.doh.goc.uk/cancer

NHS 2001 Primary care, general practice and the NHS Plan. Department of Health, London

Turner P et al 1986 Clinical pharmacology, 5th edn. Churchill Livingstone, Edinburgh

Further reading

British Medical Journal (theme issue) 2001 Apoptosis: programmed cell death. 7301, June

Caldas C 1998 Molecular assessment of cancer. British Medical Journal 316:1360–1363

National Cancer Research Network (NCRN) 2003 Annual report 2002–3. Report reference AR0302. NCRN Coordinating Centre. Online. Available at: www.ncrn.org.uk/csg/briefing.htm

Tanner G 2004 Online. Available at: www.modern.nhs.uk/cancer

CHAPTER 2

Principles and ethics of clinical trials in oncology

Chapter contents

INTRODUCTION TO DRUG DEVELOPMENT

The reconfiguration of cancer research networks in the UK has allowed a potentially greater number of patients to be enrolled onto clinical trials. Increases in survival rates will occur only if more selective anticancer agents can be discovered (Connors 1996) i.e. drugs that maximise the therapeutic effect and minimise toxicity. Historically, new drug development has been based on preclinical in vitro and in vivo studies.

In vitro studies look at the anticancer properties of a new drug compound against multiple tumour cell lines. These tools also used to look at how a new drug behaves when the cell line has specific genetic properties, such as mutations in the tumour suppressor gene p53 and expression of multidrug resistance proteins. The use of cell line panels allows evaluation of new drugs that target a specific genetic property of the tumour cell. It is now possible to determine if a given drug is likely to inhibit drug resistant tumours or kill cells that overexpress specific oncogenes at an early phase of drug discovery (Curt 1996).

This process may result in the evaluation of drugs that have anticancer activity but it requires clinical human trials to determine whether there is significant activity and acceptable toxicity. This process has been accelerated through rational drug design using, for example, X-ray crystallography and designing active drug compounds based on the crystal structure of the target. In vivo animal studies are used to study drug toxicology and drug activity against predetermined cancer cell lines. Toxicology data from preclinical in vivo studies are used to derive the starting dose for Phase I studies. Before a drug is administered to a patient, however, all the data on this drug from the preclinical in vivo and in vitro studies need to be collated and presented to the regulatory and licensing bodies, and ethical approval needs to be sought to proceed with the clinical trial. The regional ethics committee should approve the study.

NEW DRUGS REGULATORY BODIES

CLINICAL TRIAL CONTROL IN EUROPE

Cancer Phase I trials in the UK are conducted either directly by drug companies or under the auspices of the **Cancer UK Phase I/II Clinical Trials Committee**. The licence for use of a new drug in the UK is obtained through the **Medicines and Healthcare Products Regulatory Agency (MHRA)**.

The **UK Medicines Act** came into force in 1971, having been granted royal assent in 1968. At the same time, a new committee – called the **Committee on Safety of Medicines (CSM)** – was established. The purpose of the Medicines Act was to coordinate the control of the manufacture and distribution of medicines in the UK. The Act's legislative and legal powers ensured that it was illegal to manufacture and sell products that did not have the necessary licences. In 1995, the UK legislation was brought into line with that of the European Community (EC) in the marketing of medicinal products. The MHRA, as the 'licensing authority', is accountable to parliament through Health and Agriculture Ministers. Various advisory bodies make recommendations to the MHRA on a wide range of issues relating to new and established compounds.

The **Medicines Commission** was set up in 1968 by the Medicines Act. The purpose of this body is to advise Ministers on matters relating to the Medicines Act relating to medicinal products.

Once the licence and ethical approval is obtained, a study can begin. It is obligatory to obtain written consent from all patients taking part in the study.

The **Medicines for Human Use Clinical Trials Regulations** 2004 (UK and Europe) (www.hmso.gov.uk/si/si2004/20041031.htm) are now in force and already having a major impact on how clinical trials are coordinated and run in Europe; they implement the European Directive on Clinical Trials (2001/20/EC). The regulations cover patient factors such as what constitutes informed consent for patients entering a clinical trial. Investigators wanting to run a clinical trial have to ensure that there is approval from the regulatory authority of that country and from the manufacturer receiving authorisation and there is also ethical approval for the trial. There will need to be one or more sponsors of the trial to ensure that the regulations are being followed and that there is indemnity for liability covering both the sponsor and investigator. The definition of what is meant by 'conducting a clinical trial' under this Act means prescribing, directing or administering an investigational product, carrying out any procedure, or performing any test or analysis to study the clinical toxicology, pharmacology and pharmacodynamic effects of the study agent. The principles of good clinical practice (GCP) and good manufacturing practice (GMP) dictate and drive the principles of standards for starting up and conducting clinical trials.

EudraCT – the Community Clinical Trial System – is a database of all interventional clinical trials of medicinal products in the European Community. It was set up in accordance with Directive 2001/20/EC. It applies to clinical trials where both the submission to the Ethics Committee and to the Competent Authority occurs on or after 1 May 2004.

The activities of the **European Medicines Evaluation Agency** (www.emea.eu.int/pdfs/general/direct/emeaar/000204en.pdf) include the evaluation of new medicinal products for human and animal use, and scientific appraisal of new products that are submitted for use throughout the European Union. It also supervises the pharmacovigilance of licensed products and receives reports about drug adverse effects from both within and outside the European Union.

CLINICAL TRIAL CONTROL IN THE USA

The National Research Act created the Commission for the Protection of Human Subjects in Biomedical and Behavioural Research in 1974, which produced guidelines (The Belmont Report 1979) on how ethical research should be done. Federal bodies known as institutional review boards (IRBs) assess applications for research. They are in turn required to report to the Office of Human Research Protection as part of the Department of Health and Human Services. The IRBs are responsible for ensuring the proper running of clinical research, including the recording and monitoring of significant events through research such as drug toxicity. It is the responsibility of the principal investigator to conduct a 'proper' piece of clinical research or trial. The US Food and Drug Administration (FDA) is the regulatory authority for medicinal products, reviews clinical research and maintains pharmacovigilance.

INFORMED CONSENT

The purpose of informed consent is to help protect patients taking part in clinical trials and medical research. To be comprehensive, the patient must be informed about the purpose of the trial, the potential benefits and disadvantage or risks of the trial, and what interventions are likely. Patient information leaflets will need to be provided. To ensure that the information available to the patient about the trial is clear, valid and contains all pertinent information the ethics committee usually screen these when ethical approval for the study is sought. Patients must also be informed about all available treatment options. A consent form signed and dated by both the investigator and the patient is a necessary requirement. The patient, once enrolled onto the trial, has the right to leave the study at any point and is under no obligation to complete the study. The investigator must ensure that, as the trial is proceeding, any relevant information about the results of the trial is given to the patient.

ETHICAL APPROVAL

The new clinical trials regulations for the UK came into force in May 2004. They stipulate that ethical approval is required for studies that include:

- Phase I studies with healthy volunteers
- patients and users of the NHS
- relatives and carers of patients of the NHS
- where there is a need for access to biological material, e.g. tissues sample
- use of NHS access.

Research ethics committees are independent committees and at least one-third of the committee membership is defined as lay members. Lay members are usually independent of the NHS and do not have a specific specialist research interest. Local research ethics committees assess potential clinical trials within their geographical area. The governance framework to which the research ethics committees work is defined by the Department of Health Research Governance Ethics Framework (www.dh/gov/policyandguidance/researchanddevelopment). This covers a wide range of ethical issues, including human rights, patient information and confidentiality issues, the Data Protection Act and research using human tissue. The Gene Therapy Advisory Committee (GTAC) is the ethics committee for studies involving gene therapy research in humans.

Before a clinical trial takes place it *must* be approved by a research ethics committee. If a study will need to recruit across more than four centres then an application must be made to a multicentre research ethics committee. For multicentre trials within one geographical area, the application must be made to the local research ethics committee. If the clinical trial will be using an investigational medicinal product then it is compulsory for the trial to be registered through the Central Office of Research Ethics Committees (COREC; www.corec.org.uk).

COREC's role is to coordinate the work of the research ethical committees and to act as a training resource, providing training and advice to anyone involved in research. It also publishes reviews and guidance on how to make an application. A standard ethics application form is available from COREC. The ethics form appears on the COREC website, is downloadable, and is in two sections. The first section, comprising parts A–C, apply to generic information as well as the site information; part D is an optional section applying to research and development units.

Multicentre studies need to apply through the COREC central allocation system. The new regulations state that the research ethical committee must reach a decision within 60 days. The investigators can attend the research ethical committees meeting.

Before proceeding with a Phase I trial, the two key items needed are: (i) approval from a recognised Phase I research ethics committee ('recognised' means known to COREC; the application can be made directly to the research ethics committee rather than through COREC); and (ii) clinical trials authorisation (CTA) from the Medicines and Healthcare Products Regulatory Agency (MHRA).

The Department of Health and the Medical Research Council have put together a clinical trials toolkit to help researchers to formulate the paperwork necessary to meet the regulatory requirements. This is available at: www.ct-toolkit.ac.uk.

PHASE I CLINICAL TRIALS

The focus of Phase I clinical trials is to:

- judge the optimal dosing schedules for a new drug
- assess the clinical pharmacology, pharmacokinetics and pharmacodynamic effects of the drug
- determine the toxicity profile.

Clinical pharmacokinetic studies aim to determine how plasma levels of the drug relate to the pharmacodynamic effect of the drug as well as evaluating the way a drug is metabolised and excreted. Metabolites may be produced that might have anticancer activity or toxic effects on the patients.

Conventionally one of the primary aims of a Phase I trial is to determine the maximum tolerated dose (MTD) and the dose recommended for Phase II trials. However, for targeted therapies to optimal biological dose, based on pharmacological data, and not the MTD may be used to define the Part II dose. The Phase II dose is achieved through dose escalations, which are determined through observed toxicities, pharmacokinetic analysis and pharmacodynamic studies relating drug effect and toxicity to drug exposure (AUC). Phase I trials usually involve patients who have failed on previous treatment regimens and who may be heavily pretreated. The trials usually involve small numbers of patients being treated at each dose level, with the total number of patients involved being around 30 on average. Patients are selected based on strict eligibility criteria.

It is essential that the correct procedures are followed for enrolling someone onto a Phase I clinical trial. When setting up the study it is important to define the purpose of the Phase I trial, as discussed above. In addition, evidence of antitumour activity is usually needed; however, significant responses are rarely seen in Phase I trials because patients tend to have been heavily pretreated and have advanced disease.

Patient eligibility criteria should be clearly defined. For example, a proven (histological) diagnosis of a malignant disease and recovery from any prior treatment regimen. No chemotherapy or radiotherapy should be given 4–6 weeks prior to entry onto a Phase I clinical study and, if myelosuppression is a predicted toxicity, patients will be excluded from the trial if there is evidence of bone marrow infiltration or if the bone marrow is compromised by previous treatment. Eligible patients must have a reasonable level of physical and mental well-being and the World Health Organization (WHO) performance status (see Table 2.2) is used as a measure. Patients who are acutely unwell will not be considered for entry. Patients must be able to receive and understand informed consent about the implications and purpose of the clinical study. The majority of studies also have some sort of age range with a reasonable life expectancy of around 3 months. Pretreatment haematological and biochemical factors are taken into account, particularly if preclinical studies predict toxicity. Patients are excluded from the trial if they need treatment that might affect the way the study drug works or if interactions with the new drug's metabolic pathways are predicted.

Once the trial is underway, monitoring of the trial both by the internal investigators and external monitors will ensure that patients are assessed before each treatment course and that toxicity is recorded, usually using criteria such as the common toxicity criteria. The starting dose in a Phase I trial is based on the preclinical data. Dose escalation follows. Measurement of drug level and pharmacokinetic modelling of the data, together with metabolic studies, inform the investigators as to the metabolism and excretion of the drug and of the presence of active metabolites that might confer an increased risk of toxicity.

Consideration of the eligibility and exclusion criteria helps in the ethical debate of whether a patient should be offered an experimental treatment. The eligibility and exclusion criteria give an assessment on the quality of life of the patient. It should be made clear to the cancer patient that only an average 10–20% of patients at most are likely to respond clinically to a new drug undergoing Phase I clinical trials. Many of these patients see the treatment as a last chance before succumbing to their disease. Hence the decision to enrol on to such trials should be taken with full discussion within the multidisciplinary team members including the palliative care team and the GP, as well as family members. Although some of the scientific evidence might not be relevant in terms of the description of the new drug under consideration, there is a clear role for an interface between the cancer centre and primary care so that a patient's GP is aware of the purpose of the trial, what may be expected in terms of potential side effects and what impact the trial is likely to have on the quality of life of the cancer patient. Performance status is used as an eligibility criterion for most, if not all, clinical trials in cancer therapy and there are various measures that are used (see p. 27).

The development of new cancer drugs, with greater selectivity, will hopefully lead to experimental therapy being given with less toxicity and a greater likelihood of objective response. With this in mind, a study by Roberts et al (2004) looked at the trends in the rates of treatment-related death, objective response and serious toxicity in 213 Phase I trials performed over a 12-year period. They found that the level of risk experienced by cancer patients who participate in Phase I treatment trials appeared to have improved because toxic death rates have decreased more quickly than have objective response rates. Hence the risk:benefit ratio has also improved as a result perhaps better monitoring of these patients through trials.

PHASE II TRIALS

These trials use doses and schedules based on Phase I data. The aim of Phase II trials are usually to determine efficacy based on tumour response. The studies select patients with specific tumour types and each trial assesses response.

Drugs that enter Phase II trials are those that have gone through preclinica in vitro and in vivo studies and Phase I trials. Less than 10% of drugs entering Phase I trials have been shown to have clinical activity. Phase II trials usually involve a study of the activity of a single agent drug against specific tumour types and the aim is to determine how effective these drugs are.

The study design will determine how many patients need to be enrolled onto a Phase II trial; most trials recruit around 50 patients. Patients are entered onto Phase II trials if they match the eligibility criteria and maybe chemotherapy naïve. When looking at response rates, it is essential that the patients enrolled onto a Phase II trial have measurable disease.

PHASE III TRIALS

Phase III trials are full-scale evaluations of the drug involving randomisation, control groups, different study populations and different treatment protocols. Those agents that go on to Phase III have usually demonstrated activity in Phase II. The gold standards of clinical trials are a good randomised trial, which looks at new treatment compared against standard treatment for a specific cancer. The two study groups should be randomised to be comparable and selection bias minimised. Stratification may be needed to balance-out patient factors such as extent of disease that might affect response. There must be sufficient power to determine the predetermined target difference between the two groups. This may mean recruiting large numbers of patients so that the differences between the two groups can be detected; this normally involves multicentre trials.

Measure of effect is usually to use overall survival as a primary endpoint. Survival curves are produced using the Kaplan–Meir method and hazard ratios determine the degree of difference between the treatments. Other endpoints that are measured are disease-free survival and time to progression. Quality of life analysis is usually also required in these trials.

MEASURING TREATMENT RESPONSE

To make clinical trials outcome data more standardised, a new system of measuring response to treatment based on measurements of tumour size using imaging techniques was devised. The Response Evaluation Criteria in Solid Tumours (RECIST; Therasse et al 2000) guidelines were produced as collaboration between the National Cancer Institute and EORTC. These differ from the previously used WHO criteria in that unidimensional

TABLE 2.1 WHO and RECIST guidelines for the evaluation of solid tumours

Response	WHO*	RECIST*
Complete	No disease	No disease
Partial response	50% decrease	30% decrease
Stable disease	Neither partial nor progressive	Neither partial nor progressive
Progressive disease	25% increase	20% increase

* RECIST uses sum of longest diameters whereas the WHO evaluation uses the product of longest diameter and the greatest perpendicular diameter.

measurements are used. The differences between the RECIST guidelines and WHO in the evaluation of solid tumours are listed in Table 2.1.

Clinical trials state the endpoints of the trial in their protocols and also what outcomes are important. Some trials are geared towards quality of life issues whereas the majority of Phase III trials assess disease-free survival, progression-free survival and overall survival. Disease-free survival is the time between entry into a trial and the onset of recurrent disease; progression-free survival is the time between the end of treatment and the development of progressive disease or death, in adjuvant studies the term used is 'relapse-free' survival; overall survival is the time interval between entry into the trial and death from any cause.

STATISTICAL DESIGN OF PHASE III TRIALS

The aim in the design and analysis of a randomised controlled trial is to reduce bias in patient selection between the groups under study and also to have predefined which outcome data should be used in the analysis. Phase II trials are uncontrolled or open trials because there is usually only the one treatment group. In Phase II cancer trials, the usual aim is to assess the efficacy and toxicity of a new drug in cancers that might be sensitive to the compound. This will be a best guess based on the results of earlier preclinical studies and on the results of the Phase I trial. The gold standard of a randomised, double-blind, controlled study in Phase III trials is difficult when one is comparing chemotherapy agents. In making a comparison between two drugs and drug regimens it is important that the allocation of patients to treatment is unbiased, and this is usually done by random allocation. The purpose here is to balance the treatment arm against the control arm in terms of patient factors, e.g. previous treatment, age, stage of tumour. The advantage of stratified randomisation is that if it is known that there are patient prognostic variables that might affect outcome then this could be incorporated in the design and allocation of patients to various arms of the study. In less common cancers, where patient recruitment may be a problem, the process of minimisation is used to balance the arms of the trials. The minimisation process relies on looking at each new patient entered in the trial and determining which treatment the patient should receive to balance the groups in terms of patient characteristics and prognostic factors. Randomisation using a weighting factor is used to allocate patients to one of the treatment arms. Variations in the allocation of patients during randomised trials include cross-over trials in which the same groups of patients receive all the treatments available in order. There are some disadvantages, such as patient drop-outs before cross-over. Using this methodology, it is important that there is no carry-over in terms of treatment effect. When determining the number of patients to allocate to each arm of the trial, it is important that an appropriate calculation is done on the number of patients who will need to be recruited. This is the power calculation, which defines the probability that a study of a given size would detect as statistically significant a real difference of a given magnitude.

In the analyses and reporting of the trial results, the initial analysis would look at the baseline characteristics of the patients in the groups allocated to ensure that the randomisation process had balanced the groups, e.g. for prognostic variables. The main analysis of the data looks at the different groups against the prestated outcome measures. The type of statistical analysis depends on the type of data available for analysis. The data should be analysed on an intention-to-treat basis so that the treatment groups are balanced, reducing bias and taking into account patients who might have dropped out of the trial for various reasons. All patients should be accounted for. The aim is to report the number of patients who completed therapy, those who died or who were not eligible, those lost to follow-up and the length of follow-up. The analysis and reporting of interim results is important and, when there is an early termination of a trial, a full explanation of why patients were not recruited further is needed.

In trials with multiple outcome measures, a correction might need to be made to the P value (a measure of statistical significance) to take this into account. The danger of doing subgroup analyses (analysing the data available as different subsets of data) is that the statistical analyses might not match clinical efficacy, particularly if the subsets are small. A common alternative method of analysis is a meta-analysis, in which data from several published trials are analysed together. An evaluation is made not only of all relevant trials but also the quality of the trials. The risk with meta-analyses is that of publication bias, whereby trials that show negative or no response to treatment are less likely to be published. Similarly, different trials may be too heterogeneous to compare. This may complicate their inclusion in a single analysis.

QUALITY OF LIFE MEASUREMENTS AND PERFORMANCE STATUS

Increasingly, cancer trials are looking at quality of life issues when assessing the health status of patients who are proceeding through chemotherapy. Health-related quality of life (HRQL) is a measure of how cancer and cancer treatment impacts on the patient. The instruments used to measure HRQL are usually questionnaires comprising a series of questions that, in turn, are combined to form a domain or dimension of an area of measurable behaviour (Guyatt 1993). This can be done through interviews through telephone consultation or by self-recording. The power of any HRQL questionnaire relies on how discriminative it is; it must be possible to tell the difference in quality of life between two people. Various methods are used to construct and determine if a HRQL questionnaire is reliable. The questions that are used can be disease specific and relate to both physical and mental well-being, as well as to side effects of treatment. Studies looking at the use of new chemotherapy regimens are well placed to look at the trade-off between the length of time of remission and quality of life.

Many types of instrument have been used to measure quality of life, including the Functional Living Index – Cancer, the Quality of Life Index, the Functional Assessment of Cancer Therapy – General, the Cancer Rehabilitation Evaluation System and the Quality of Life Questionnaire – Cancer.

The Quality of Life Group (www.eortc.be/home/qol), which is part of EORTC, coordinates and advises on the design and analysis of quality of life studies within Phase III trials. The EORTC QLQ-C30 is a questionnaire instrument used to assess the quality of life of cancer patients (Fig. 2.1). It has been used in worldwide trials and disease-specific modules have been used in diseases such as breast and lung cancer.

PERFORMANCE STATUS

Performance status is used in practically all clinical cancer drug trials to give a surrogate measure of the quality of life of patients being considered for treatment; it is also a prognostic variable. It has been shown that patients with poor performance status are less likely to complete treatment and have much poorer outcomes, although functional status and overall quality of life show weaker correlation. Three widely used measures of performance scales are the:

- Eastern Cooperative Oncology Group (ECOG) scale
- World Health Organization (WHO) scales
- Karnofsky performance scores.

EORTC QLQ-C30 (version 3)   Specimen

We are interested in some things about you and your health. Please answer all of the questions yourself by circling the number that best applies to you. There are no 'right' or 'wrong' answers. The information that you provide will remain strictly confidential.

Please fill in your initials:

Your birthdate (Day, Month, Year):

Today's date (Day, Month, Year):

	Not at all	A little	Quite a bit	Very much
1. Do you have any trouble doing strenuous activities, like carrying a heavy shopping bag or a suitcase?	1	2	3	4
2. Do you have any trouble taking a <u>long</u> walk?	1	2	3	4
3. Do you have any trouble taking a <u>short</u> walk outside of the house?	1	2	3	4
4. Do you need to stay in bed or a chair during the day?	1	2	3	4
5. Do you need help with eating, dressing, washing yourself or using the toilet?	1	2	3	4

During the past week:	Not at all	A little	Quite a bit	Very much
6. Were you limited in doing either your work or other daily activities?	1	2	3	4
7. Were you limited in pursuing your hobbies or other leisure time activities?	1	2	3	4
8. Were you short of breath?	1	2	3	4
9. Have you had pain?	1	2	3	4
10. Did you need rest?	1	2	3	4
11. Have you had trouble sleeping?	1	2	3	4
12. Have you felt weak?	1	2	3	4
13. Have you lacked appetite?	1	2	3	4
14. Have you felt nauseated?	1	2	3	4
15. Have you vomited?	1	2	3	4
16. Have you been constipated?	1	2	3	4

Fig. 2.1 Examples from the QLQ-C30 (reproduced with the permission of the EORTC Quality of Life Study Group).

During the past week:	Not at all	A little	Quite a bit	Very much
17. Have you had diarrhea?	1	2	3	4
18. Were you tired?	1	2	3	4
19. Did pain interfere with your daily activities?	1	2	3	4
20. Have you had difficulty in concentrating on things, like reading a newspaper or watching television?	1	2	3	4
21. Did you feel tense?	1	2	3	4
22. Did you worry?	1	2	3	4
23. Did you feel irritable?	1	2	3	4
24. Did you feel depressed?	1	2	3	4
25. Have you had difficulty remembering things?	1	2	3	4
26. Has your physical condition or medical treatment interfered with your family life?	1	2	3	4
27. Has your physical condition or medical treatment interfered with your social activities?	1	2	3	4
28. Has your physical condition or medical treatment caused you financial difficulties?	1	2	3	4

For the following questions please circle the number between 1 and 7 that best applies to you

29. How would you rate your overall health during the past week?

1	2	3	4	5	6	7
Very poor						Excellent

30. How would you rate your overall quality of life during the past week?

1	2	3	4	5	6	7
Very poor						Excellent

Fig. 2.1 *Continued*

ECOG performance status (Table 2.2)

World Health Organization (WHO) scale for performance status (Table 2.3)

Karnofsky scores

The Karnofsky performance scores are widely used measures of quality of life with functional status, which is a measure of response to treatment and is another measure that can give a prognostic indication of how well patients may do (Table 2.4). The Karnofsky scores suffer from being a measure of physical functioning rather than of the non-physical measures relating to social and emotional aspects of health and a cross-validation study with the EORTC QLQ-30 suggested that these factors should also be assessed during cancer care of patients with advanced disease (Schaafsma 1994).

TABLE 2.2 ECOG performance status (with permission)

Grade	Description
0	Fully active, able to carry out all predisease performance without restriction
1	Restricted in physically strenuous activity but ambulatory and able to carry out work of a light or sedentary nature, e.g. light housework, office work
2	Ambulatory and capable of all self-care but unable to carry out any work activities. Up and about more than 50% of waking hours
3	Capable of only limited self-care, confined to bed or chair more than 50% of waking hours
4	Completely disabled, cannot carry on any self-care. Totally confined to bed or chair
5	Dead

TABLE 2.3 WHO scale for performance status

Grade	Description
0	Fully active, able to carry on all predisease performance without restriction
1	Restricted in physically strenuous activity but ambulatory and able to carry out work of a light or sedentary nature, e.g. light housework, office work
2	Ambulatory and capable of self-care but unable to carry out any work activities. Up and about more than 50% of waking hours
3	Capable of only limited self-care, confined to bed or chair more than 50% of waking hours
4	Completely disabled. Cannot carry out any self-care. Totally confined to bed or chair
5	Dead

TABLE 2.4 The Karnofsky performance scores

Score	Description
100	Normal
90	Normal activity, minor symptoms
80	Normal activity with some symptoms
70	Self-caring: cannot do active work
60	Able to self-care but requires some assistance
50	Needs medical care and a lot of assistance
40	Needs special care and disabled
30	Needs to be hospitalised
20	Very unwell, death not imminent
10	Moribund, progressing

PHASE IV

Phase IV studies involve postmarketing surveillance. The Committee on Safety of Medicines (CSM) – one of the independent advisory committees established under the Medicines Act – advises the UK Licensing Authority on the quality, efficacy and safety of medicines. The Committee's role is to advise the Licensing Authority on whether new medicinal products submitted to the UK MHRA should be granted marketing rights in collaboration with the MHRA's Licensing Division. The MHRA's Post-Licensing Division works with the CSM to make sure that safety and efficacy issues relating to a product are maintained.

The **yellow card scheme** (the yellow cards are found in the back of the *British National Formulary*) is a mechanism through which the CSM (centrally or regionally) receives reports of adverse drug effects associated with a new or an established drug. It relies on voluntary reporting and applies not only to doctors but to nurses, dentists, pharmaceutical companies and pharmacists.

The **black triangle symbol** against a product entry in the *British National Formulary*, *MIMS* and *ABPI Compendium of Datasheets and Summaries of Product Characteristics* indicates that the CSM, in tandem with the postlicensing division of the MRHA, is monitoring the new medicinal product; this monitoring lasts for a minimum 2-year period. The criteria as to when the black triangle is assigned apply to a new drug, a combination of drugs, when an existing product is given by a new route or drug delivery system, and where the drug is given for a new indication.

The MRHA assesses the adverse drug reactions reported on the yellow cards, looking at associated factors such as concurrent medication that might have resulted in the reactions. A drug can be withdrawn if safety is compromised over efficacy. An example of this was the withdrawal of rofecoxib, a COX II inhibitor that was found to cause sudden death in susceptible groups. Alternatively, the side effect might simply be listed in the product literature or the licence altered for particular groups, exempting other patient groups who may be susceptible to adverse drug reactions.

References/further reading

Belmont Report 1979 The National Commission for the Protection of Human Subjects of Biomedical and Behavioural Research. Washington DC

Connors T 1996 Anticancer drug development: the way forward. The Oncologist 1(3):180–181

Curt GA 1996 Cancer drug development: new targets for cancer treatment. The Oncologist 1(3):120-ii–120-iii

Guyatt GH et al 1993 Measuring health-related quality of life. Annals of Internal Medicine 118:622–629

Roberts TG 2004 Trends in the risks and benefits to patients with cancer participating in phase 1 clinical trials. Journal of the American Medical Association 292(17):2130–2140

Schaafsma J, Osoba D 1994 The Karnofsky Performance Status scale re-examined: a cross-validation with the EORTC-C30. Quality of Life Research 3(6):413–424

Therasse P et al 2000 New guidelines to evaluate the response to treatment in solid tumours. Journal of the National Cancer Institute 92(3):205–216

CHAPTER 3

Classification and principles of use of anticancer drugs

INTRODUCTION

This chapter discusses drugs that are already available in clinical practice for cancer treatment; the role of agents such as antiangiogenic drugs, matrix metalloproteinase inhibitors, cancer vaccines and gene therapy will be discussed separately in Chapter 6.

   Anticancer drugs can be classified as follows:

- Hormonal agents:
  - steroids
  - aromatase inhibitors
  - antiandrogens
  - luteinising hormone-releasing hormone (LHRH) analogues
  - oestrogen-receptor antagonists
  - progestogens
  - somatostatin analogues.
- Biological modifiers:
  - interferons
  - interleukins
  - colony stimulating factors
  - monoclonal antibodies
  - non-specific immunomodulating drugs.

- Cytotoxic drugs:
  - alkylators
  - antimetabolites
  - antibiotics/anthracyclines
  - Tubulin binding drugs, plant derived – vinca alkaloids and taxanes
  - topoisomerase I and II inhibitors.

ANTI-HORMONAL THERAPY

A range of common cancers that are responsive to the effect of hormonal manipulation can be treated by hormonal therapy. The range of use of hormonal therapy includes the adjuvant and neoadjuvant setting, primary and secondary prevention and treatment and palliation in advanced disease. Table 3.1 classifies the more common types of endocrine therapy used.

A hormone is a chemical substance secreted by an endocrine gland. It will have an effect on an organ(s) or tissue(s) elsewhere in the body, either in proximity or distal to the gland that produced it. For a hormone to exert its effect it requires an extracellular transport system, and usually attaches to plasma proteins to enable it to reach the target tissue. At the target tissue the hormone could attach to intracellular receptors. It enters the cell it binds to its receptor, which in turn results in intracellular activation of a protein complex, leading to a net target effect.

TABLE 3.1 Classification of hormonal agents used in the treatment and palliation of cancers

Type of agent	Example drugs
Steroids	Corticosteroids
Aromatase inhibitors	Exemestane (steroidal) Anastrozole and letrozole (non-steroidal)
Antiandrogens	Flutamide, biclutamide, cyproterone acetate
LHRH analogues	Leuprorelin, goserelin, buserelin
Oestrogen-receptor antagonists	Diethylstilboestrol, tamoxifen, fulvestrant, toremifene
Progestogens	Medroxyprogesterone acetate, megestrol acetate, norethisterone
Somatostatin analogues	Octreotide

LHRH, luteinising hormone-releasing hormone.

Hormones and cell effect:

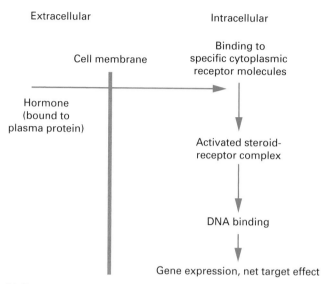

Fig. 3.1 Diagrammatic representation of how a hormonal drug bound to plasma protein crosses the cell membrane to bind to intracellular specific receptors, causing a net target effect.

Many agents have been developed to interfere with the interaction between the hormone molecule and its receptor; an interaction that stimulates cell growth and proliferation. Perhaps the best example, the antioestrogen drug tamoxifen acts by attaching to oestrogen receptors within the cytoplasm. This blocks initiation (by the hormone oestrogen) of the intracellular processes that normally lead to proliferation. By blocking the action of oestrogen at its receptor site, tamoxifen interferes with oestrogenic effects on breast cells and breast cancer cells (Fig. 3.1).

STEROIDS

Adrenal corticosteroid treatment

Steroid hormones (Table 3.2, Figs 3.2 and 3.3) bind to cytoplasmic steroid receptors. They have been used in the treatment of haematological malignancies such as myeloma, lymphomas and leukaemia. In these conditions it is thought that steroids act to increase the apoptotic response in target cells. In solid tumours such as prostate and breast cancer, the purpose

TABLE 3.2 Important organs in the biosynthesis of steroid hormones

Organ	Hormones produced
Adrenal gland	Glucocorticoids, mineralocorticoids, androgens, oestrogens, progesterone
Ovaries	Androgens and oestrogens
Testis	Androgens and oestrogens
Placenta	Progesterone and oestrogens
Corpus luteum	Progesterone
Hypothalamus	Luteinising hormone-releasing hormone
Pituitary	Luteinising hormone and follicle stimulating hormone

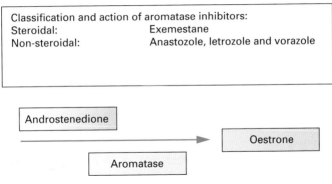

Classification and action of aromatase inhibitors:
Steroidal: Exemestane
Non-steroidal: Anastozole, letrozole and vorazole

Androstenedione → Aromatase → Oestrone

Fig. 3.2 Classification and action of aromatase inhibitors.

of using corticosteroids is to reduce tumour inflammation and oedema and palliate symptoms in advanced disease. This includes the treatment of nausea and vomiting and stimulating appetite.

The side effects of steroid treatment include a cushingoid appearance, sodium retention leading to fluid retention, hypertension, diabetes and immune suppression leading to increased risk of infection (Rutz 2002).

Aminogluthemide
This is an oral agent used as a non-steroidal inhibitor of corticosteroid synthesis. It acts as a medical adrenalectomy to reduce the synthesis of androgens, oestrogens, glucocorticoids and mineralocorticoids. The key stages of inhibition of enzymes in the production of these hormones include:

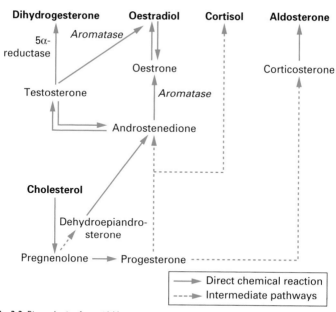

Fig. 3.3 Biosynthesis of steroidal hormones.

- inhibition of adrenal steroid synthesis, blocking conversion of cholesterol to pregnenolone
- inhibition of extra-adrenal oestradiol and oestrone synthesis
- inhibition of the aromatase enzyme that catalyses conversion of androstenedione to oestrone.

Aminogluthemide is metabolised in the liver. The toxicity of this drug means that it is not used now in cancer treatment. It requires the coadministration of hydrocortisone to prevent adrenal insufficiency (which can present as hyperkalaemia, hyponatraemia and postural hypotension) and the steroid cover needs to be increased at times of stress such as concurrent infection, trauma or at the time of surgery. Orthostatic hypotension may require fludrocortisone and symptoms of hypothyroidism may occur, hence thyroid function tests need to be performed. Severe somnolence and lethargy may occur. If a patient develops a skin rash it is usually within the first 7 days and is usually self-limiting.

Aminogluthemide interacts with drugs such as warfarin, digoxin and theophylline.

AROMATASE INHIBITORS

The peripheral conversion of androgens by aromatase, a P450 cytochrome enzyme, accounts for oestrogen production after the menopause. The two sites of production of oestrogens are within the adrenal gland and in fat. In premenopausal women the main site of production of oestrogens is in the ovary and hence oestrogen levels are not dependent on aromatase inhibitors. The aromatase inhibitors can be classed as either:

- steroidal: exemestane
- non-steroidal: anastrozole, letrozole.

In the UK anastrozole, exemestane and letrozole are licensed for use in the treatment of advanced breast cancer in postmenopausal women (Ravdin 2002). Randomised clinical trials have supported the use of the newer selective aromatase inhibitors as first-line treatment of hormone-receptor-positive metastatic breast cancer in postmenopausal women. Anastrozole also has a licence for the adjuvant treatment of oestrogen-receptor-positive early breast cancer in women unable to take tamoxifen.

Anastrozole

This is a new, selective, non-steroidal aromatase inhibitor. Unlike aminogluthemide it does not appear to have an effect on glucocorticoid or mineralocorticoid synthesis. It inhibits the conversion of adrenal androgens to oestrogens, i.e. it blocks the aromatisation of precursors to oestrogen, reducing oestrogen concentrations. Suppression of serum oestradiol levels can take 2 weeks.

Anastrozole is taken orally and is unaffected by food. The usual dose is 1 mg once daily and doses do not need to be adjusted for patients who have renal or hepatic impairment. It is metabolised within the liver and excreted in the faeces. Its main clinical use is in the treatment of advanced breast cancer as first-line treatment in postmenopausal women with either oestrogen-receptor-positive or unknown disease. It is also given to oestrogen-receptor-positive postmenopausal women who have progressed on tamoxifen therapy given in the adjuvant setting. It is given as adjuvant treatment in postmenopausal women with hormone-receptor-positive early stage breast cancer who are unable to tolerate Tamoxifen or in whom Tamoxifen is contraindicated. Patients should be warned about hot flushes, arthralgias and asthenia. It is associated with bone fractures with an increased risk of osteoporosis and trials are underway assessing the combination of bisphosphonates with anastrozole. There is a lower risk of endometrial cancer and thrombosis compared to tamoxifen.

The Arimedex, Tamoxifen Alone or in Combination (ATAC) Trial reported on the clinical effectiveness of anastrozole compared with tamoxifen as part of adjuvant therapy in breast cancer. After 33 months of follow-up in patients with oestrogen-receptor-positive breast tumours, anastrozole was significantly better than tamoxifen, reducing the risk of recurrence by 22%

and the risk of developing a primary cancer in the contralateral breast by a relative 58%, which equates to a disease-free survival of 91% at 3 years compared to 89% in the tamoxifen group (ATAC Trialists Group 2002). Further follow-up is needed on the benefit of using anastrozole for 5 years, as is the case with tamoxifen. The evidence to date is that in early disease tamoxifen should be the first-line adjuvant therapy but that anastrozole is indicated for women who cannot tolerate tamoxifen.

Letrozole

This acts as a non-steroidal inhibitor of aromatase. It is metabolised in the liver by the cytochrome P450 system and hence care has to be taken with potential drug interactions. It is dosed at 2.5 mg once daily and is indicated only for postmenopausal women. Evidence from a randomised trial has suggested a use in the neoadjuvant setting: postmenopausal women with oestrogen-receptor-positive locally advanced breast cancer had higher tumour response rates compared to tamoxifen to allow breast-conserving surgery (Mouridsen et al 2003). However, more evidence is needed in this setting compared with tamoxifen. Similarly, randomised trials have shown the benefit of using letrozole in locally advanced or metastatic cancer. With a follow-up of just over 30 months, letrozole reduced disease progression and increased tumour response rate compared with tamoxifen; there was no difference in overall survival. It did appear that women who were treated with tamoxifen did less well in terms of tumour response if they had received tamoxifen, as opposed to letrozole, in the adjuvant setting (Drugs and Therapeutics Bulletin 2003).

Liver function tests should be performed prior to treatment and during therapy as elevations in serum transaminases and bilirubin have been observed.

ANDROGEN PRODUCTION/ANTIANDROGENS

Antiandrogen therapy can work in several ways to reduce circulating androgens and target organ stimulation. Inhibition of the central control of hormone production through manipulation of the hypothalamohypophyseal portal system and androgen receptors are two ways in which antiandrogen therapy works.

Testosterone production by the testis is controlled by luteinising hormone (LH), which is secreted by the pituitary gland. Testosterone production also occurs through the adrenal glands via the conversion of cholesterol to either dehydroepiandrosterone or androstenedione or through the production of progesterone, which again is converted to androstenedione.

Androstenedione and testosterone are either converted via the action of aromatase to oestrone and oestradiol or via the action of 5-reductase to dihydrotestosterone.

Antiandrogens

Bicalutamide This antiandrogen has been used in locally advanced prostate cancer. It is an antiandrogen drug that inhibits the binding of androgens to androgen receptors in androgen-sensitive prostate cancer cells. It is metabolised in the liver and has a long half-life. It is used in combination with an LHRH analogue and has an oral formulation.

Liver function tests should be monitored at baseline and throughout treatment because there might be a rise in transaminases. There is an increased procoagulant effect with warfarin. Side effects include hot flushes, impotence in over 50% of patients and constipation. It is used to reduce tumour flares with gonadotrophin analogues.

Flutamide Flutamide is an antiandrogen used in both local and advanced prostate cancer. It is administered orally and acts as a non-steroidal antiandrogen, binding to androgen receptors. It is metabolised by the cytochrome P450 system and, as a result, can inhibit metabolism of warfarin leading to an increased anticoagulant effect.

Side effects include impotence, hot flushes, gynaecomastia, decreased libido, nausea and discoloration of urine.

Cyproterone acetate

This is a progestational, competitive inhibitor that prevents binding of androgens (dihydrotestosterone) to nuclear receptors and suppresses gonadal androgen production. It also has a negative feedback effect on the hypothalamopituitary axis, by inhibiting the secretion of LH and so resulting in diminished production of testicular testosterone. Hence, in prostate cancer it works by preventing testosterone from binding to androgen receptors in the prostate gland.

Cyproterone acetate is used to block the effects of the initial tumour flare associated with LHRH analogues due to increased testosterone levels. It is given orally and is metabolised in the liver. It is associated with abnormal reduced reversible spermatogenesis. It can interact with alcohol to give a reduced antiandrogen effect as well as an increased risk of thromboembolic disease with oestrogens. It can cause fluid retention, mood changes and worsen liver function tests; liver function tests should be monitored periodically. There is an increased risk of thromboembolic disease.

LHRH ANALOGUES/GONADOTROPHIN-RELEASING HORMONE AGONISTS

Goserelin and leuprorelin acetate

These drugs are synthetic peptide analogues of gonadotrophin-releasing hormone. Their effects on the pituitary are to initially stimulate follicle stimulating hormone (FSH) and LH, and then to inhibit the production of these two hormones through negative feedback.

Goserelin and leuprorelin acetate are used in the treatment of metastatic prostate cancer and work by reducing testicular androgen synthesis, which usually occurs 2–4 weeks after initiation of treatment. The usual dose of goserelin (Zoladex®) is 3.6 mg s.c. every 28 days or 10.8 mg s.c. every 90 days. Leuprorelin (Prostap®) is given as a subcutaneous at a dose of 11.25 mg every 3 months.

Goserelin and leuprorelin acetate should be used with caution in patients with renal dysfunction. Tumour flare occurs with these drugs in up to 20% of patients within 2 weeks of the start of treatment and they should not be given to patients with impending spinal cord compression or ureteral obstruction. The use of an antiandrogen before using LHRH analogues prevents tumour flare and drugs such as cyproterone acetate and flutamide are used for this purpose.

Other side effects include gynaecomastia in up to 10% of patients, impotence and decreased libido in 20% and hot flushes in 50% of patients.

Buserelin

This drug is an LHRH agonist that causes suppression of gonadotrophin secretion. It leads to reduced secretion of LH and FSH from the pituitary and, subsequently, to low testosterone levels. In Europe it is licensed for the treatment of metastatic prostatic cancer. It is initially administered subcutaneously followed by the intranasal route. Tumour flare may occur in 20% of patients, resulting in increasing bone pain, urinary retention or spinal cord compression. This tends to occur within 2 weeks of starting therapy and an antiandrogen must be given as pretreatment. The low testosterone levels result in hot flushes, reduced libido and erectile dysfunction. Buserelin must be used with caution in patients with renal impairment.

OESTROGEN-RECEPTOR ANTAGONISTS

Diethylstilboestrol

Diethylstilboestrol is an oestrogen used in the treatment of breast and prostate cancer, although its use over the last 20 years has reduced in advanced prostate cancer because of the use of LHRH analogues. Its side effect profile includes gynaecomastia, cardiovascular toxicity including ischaemic heart disease and risk of thromboembolic disease; LHRH analogues now have a safer toxicity profile. Diethylstilboestrol has been associated with vaginal adenocarcinoma in the offspring of women who took it in pregnancy.

Tamoxifen

Tamoxifen is a competitive partial agonist–inhibitor of oestrogen function. It binds to the oestrogen receptors on malignant cells in oestrogen-sensitive tissues. Its other actions include suppressing serum insulin-like growth factor-1 and upregulating local transforming growth factor-β (TGF-β) production. It is given orally at a dose of 20 mg daily.

Tamoxifen is used in the treatment of breast cancer, and as chemoprevention in high-risk breast cancer. It is effective in both pre- and postmenopausal women with oestrogen-receptor-positive breast cancer. Tamoxifen reduces recurrence rates in this group: in the first year of use the reduction in the relative risk of recurrence is 21%, 30% for the first 2 years and 50% for 5 years; there is no additional benefit for using tamoxifen for a longer period. There is an additional 33% reduction in disease recurrence for a further 5 years after stopping tamoxifen after 5-year use, compared to women who have never received the drug. In those women without lymph node involvement, tamoxifen increases 10-year survival from 73% to 79%; it increases 10-year survival from 50% to 60% in women who do have lymph node involvement. Tamoxifen reduces the risk of breast cancer in the contralateral breast by similar figures.

Side effects include nausea, hot flushes and fluid retention and an increased risk of thrombosis. Its agonist properties means that it can increase the risk of endometrial cancer.

Toremifene

This is an antioestrogen. Its effects and toxicities are similar to tamoxifen except that there is no increased risk of endometrial cancer. It is indicated in postmenopausal women with metastatic breast cancer. The response rates are similar to those with tamoxifen. However, there does appear to be cross-resistance in that women on tamoxifen are unlikely to respond to toremifene if they develop new disease. Toremifene has been found to reduce the incidence of prostate cancer for men at high risk for the disease.

Raloxifene

This is a selective oestrogen receptor modulator. Because of its partial agonist effect it is used to lower the risk of breast cancer in postmenopausal women with osteoporosis. The STAR (Study of Tamoxifen and Raloxifene) study is now comparing tamoxifen and raloxifene in high-risk women.

Its side effects are similar to those of tamoxifen. Raloxifene does not seem to increase the risk of endometrial cancer.

Fulvestrant (Faslodex®)

This is a pure oestrogen receptor antagonist. It degrades the oestrogen receptors present in breast cancer cells. It is given as an intramuscular injection and its effects last for 1 month. It is metabolised by the liver microsomal enzymes. The majority of the drug is excreted faecally. The main side effects of treatment are flu-like symptoms, asthenia, headache and skin rashes and sore throats. It should be used with caution in patients on anticoagulation therapy and is contraindicated in pregnancy. It is used in the treatment of metastatic breast cancer in postmenopausal women with oestrogen-receptor-positive advanced disease. It is given after disease progression following antioestrogenic therapy such as tamoxifen, as there is evidence that it is effective in women who have become resistant to tamoxifen.

PROGESTOGENS

Megace

This drug is a synthetic derivative of progesterone. It has an antioestrogenic effect and also inhibits the release of LH, thus resulting in reduced oestrogen levels. It is available orally. A large proportion of the drug is metabolised in the liver; it is renally excreted. Megace has a variety of roles, including the treatment of breast and endometrial cancer, renal cell cancer and as an appetite stimulant in cancers. It has been associated with an increased risk of thromboembolic disease. It should be used with caution in patients with diabetes (hyperglycaemia) and in patients with abnormal liver function. It also leads to fluid retention and patients should be on a low salt diet. Gastrointestinal symptoms, tumour flare, hot flushes and sweating have all been reported.

SOMATOSTATIN ANALOGUES

Somatostatin is a peptide that inhibits the release of growth hormone, insulin, glucagons and gastrin. Analogues of somatostatin have long half-lives. They are octapeptides that bind to the somatostatin receptor. They are indicated for chemotherapy-induced diarrhoea, symptom control in carcinoid tumours and secretory neuroendocrine tumours. The two agents used in clinical practice are octreotide and lanreotide. Octreotide needs to be given s.c. three times a day; the longer-acting formulation can be given i.m. every 4 weeks. Lanreotide is given as an i.m injection every 2 weeks.

BIOLOGICAL RESPONSE MODIFIERS

The different types of biological response modifier are shown in Table 3.3.

INTERFERONS

Interferon-α

This form of immunotherapy works either as an antiproliferative agent or to induce an immunological cytotoxic T-cell reaction. It is given either subcutaneously or intramuscularly. It is indicated in a range of tumour types,

TABLE 3.3 The biological response modifiers

Type	Example
Interferons	Interferon-α
Interleukins	Aldesleukin
Colony stimulating factors	Erythropoietin/G-CSF/GM-CSF
Monoclonal antibodies	Alemtuzumab, rituximab, trastuzumab
Non-specific immunomodulators	Bacille Calmette–Guérin

G-CSF, granulocyte colony stimulating factor; GM-CSF, granulocyte–macrophage colony stimulating factor.

including renal cell cancers, multiple myeloma, malignant melanoma, lymphoma and chronic myelogenous leukaemia. It is excreted renally. Phenytoin and phenobarbitone levels may increase on treatment. Live vaccines are contraindicated for 3 months after interferon treatment. Toxicity includes flu-like symptoms, fatigue, neurological toxicities (including confusion and depression) myelosuppression, renal toxicity, hepatotoxicity and cardiac toxicity (hypotension, congestive cardiac failure).

INTERLEUKINS

Aldesleukin (recombinant interleukin-2)

Aldesleukin is an immunomodulator that binds to interleukin-2 receptors to activate lymphokines and γ-interferon. It is usually given subcutaneously and is eliminated through the kidneys. It has a licence in the UK for use in metastatic renal cell cancer but has also been used for the treatment of malignant melanoma. Patients are at risk of capillary leak syndrome, which leads to hypotension, effusions, ascites and cognitive impairment that is made worse with the use of NSAIDs. It is nephrotoxic and reversibly hepatotoxic. Patients usually report flu-like illness and may develop skin rashes. Myelosuppression can occur.

COLONY STIMULATING FACTORS

Erythropoietin

This colony stimulating factor results in increased division and differentiation of red blood cells in the bone marrow. It is produced through recombinant DNA techniques and is given either intravenously or, more commonly, subcutaneously in the community. It is used to treat chemotherapy-induced anaemia and anaemia associated with chronic renal failure, and also to increase autologous blood prior to surgery.

Two forms are available: epoetin-α and epoetin-β. Darbepoetin is a derivative of epoetin and has a longer half-life, necessitating less frequent administration. The Committee on Safety of Medicines has issued a warning about the risk of red cell aplasia in patients treated with epoetin-α. If this complication occurs then the drug must be discontinued and testing for erythropoietin antibodies are indicated. These patients should not receive erythropoietin again.

Epoetin-α and epoetin-β should not be given to patients with uncontrolled blood pressure or those allergic to human albumin. Blood counts should be done weekly on treatment, with increases in haemoglobin (Hb) seen after 7 days of therapy. The aim is to increase Hb concentration not more than 2 g/100 mL per month, maintaining Hb at a level of 10–12 g/100 mL. If the haematocrit rises to above 40%, the dose of erythropoietin should be stopped until it falls to 35%. A dose reduction is needed by 25% on restarting treatment. If there is no response to treatment after 4–8 weeks then the dose of erythropoietin could be increased. Side effects include the possibility of dose-dependent increases in blood pressure in rare instances leading to hypertensive crisis with encephalopathy, gastrointestinal upset with diarrhoea and nausea and vomiting. Flu-like symptoms have been reported.

Granulocyte colony stimulating factor (filgrastim or lenograstim) and granulocyte–macrophage colony stimulating factor

These cytokines increase the pool of circulating neutrophils by stimulating myeloid precursors; this process occurs within 1 day of administration. If a patient has an episode of febrile neutropenia or prolonged neutropenia then the initial modification to treatment would be dose reductions and/or delaying chemotherapy. However, reductions in doses have shown to lead to an adverse outcome through clinical trials. Granulocyte colony stimulating factor (G-CSF) and granulocyte–macrophage colony stimulating factor (GM-CSF) can be used to avoid multiple dose reductions or delays. They are not usually used in primary prophylaxis after standard-dose chemotherapy for solid tumours. They are used to facilitate an increase in intensity.

Both cytokines have been used to support high-dose chemotherapy regimens in randomised controlled trials. Further work is necessary to define the best dose and scheduling regimens for G-CSF and GM-CSF.

They are given subcutaneously and the main side effects associated with treatment include pain at the site of the injection, headache, wheeze, weight gain, palpitations and chest pain.

MONOCLONAL ANTIBODIES

Alemtuzumab (Campath®)

This is a recombinant monoclonal antibody that acts against the cell surface glycoprotein CD52, which is expressed on malignant B and T lymphocytes. It is used in relapsed and/or refractory B-cell chronic lymphocytic leukaemia

(B-CLL). Patients should already have received alkylating agents and have failed fludarabine therapy.

Alemtuzumab is given as an intravenous formulation. Infusion-related reactions occur and patients usually receive premedication. These patients are at risk of immunosuppression and myelosuppression, and a greater risk of opportunistic infections.

Rituximab

This monoclonal antibody targets the CD20 glycoprotein that causes lysis of B lymphocytes. The National Institute for Clinical Excellence (NICE) has recommended this drug for use in follicular non-Hodgkin's lymphoma (stage III or IV) if patients have already failed other treatments or are intolerant. It is also used for aggressive non-Hodgkin's B-cell lymphoma (stages II–IV) in combination chemotherapy.

It is given intravenously. It requires premedication to lower the risk of infusion-related reactions, and fatalities have been documented. Patients are at risk of cardiotoxicity, skin reactions and tumour lysis syndrome.

Trastuzumab

This drug is a recombinant humanised monoclonal antibody directed against HER-2/neu human epidermal growth factor; this receptor is expressed in up to 30% of breast cancers. The mechanism of action includes an immunologically mediated reaction that includes cell lysis leading to apoptosis. If patients' tumours express HER-2/neu then trastuzumab is indicated in metastatic breast cancer as first-line therapy in combination with paclitaxel. It is also given as second- and third-line therapy as a single agent. Women with oestrogen-receptor-positive tumours should have received hormonal therapy. Trastuzumab is given as an i.v. loading dose followed by maintenance dose i.v. on a weekly basis. Infusion-related side effects including flu-like symptoms, bronchospasm and hypotension may occur in up to 50% of patients. It may cause cardiotoxicity leading to breathlessness, dependent oedema with impaired left ventricular function. This toxicity increases with the use of combination chemotherapy with the taxanes or with anthracyclines. Anthracyclines should be avoided and delayed use of trastuzumab should be considered if there has been recent use of an anthracycline (even up to 22 weeks). Pulmonary toxicity including infiltrates and pleural effusions may occur. Myelosuppression may be severe.

NON-SPECIFIC IMMUNOMODULATORS

Bacille Calmette–Guérin

This drug originates from an attenuated strain of *Mycobacterium bovis*. It is indicated for use in superficial transitional cell cancer of the bladder either as primary tumour or as recurrence leading to an inflammatory reaction in the bladder. The response appears to be immune mediated. It is usually given intravesically on a weekly basis following an induction course. It is contraindicated in patients on immunosuppressive therapy and those on antibiotics such as the quinolones, which affect the activity of the bacille Calmette–Guérin (BCG); it is also contraindicated when there is an active urinary tract infection. Side effects include a chemical cystitis with dysuria and haematuria, flu-like symptoms and gastrointestinal toxicity.

CLASSIFICATION OF CYTOTOXIC DRUGS

Cytotoxic drugs are potentially toxic drugs that should be administered only through the cancer units and centres and under specialist care. There are strict guidelines on the handling of cytotoxic drugs and the administration of drugs for intrathecal use. The classification below covers the more common cytotoxic drugs that have been used in standard regimens in the treatment of cancer:

- Alkylators and platinum drugs:
  - BCNU
  - busulphan
  - carboplatin
  - cisplatin
  - chlorambucil
  - cyclophosphamide
  - dacarbazine
  - hexamethylamine
  - ifosfamide
  - mechlorethamine
  - melphalan
  - mitomycin-C
  - oxaliplatin
  - procarbazine
  - thiotepa.
- Antimetabolites:
  - 5-fluorouracil
  - capecitabine
  - methotrexate
  - gemcitabine
  - hydroxyurea
  - 6-MP
  - ralitrexed.

- Antibiotics:
  - doxorubicin hydrochloride (epirubicin and daunorubicin)
  - DaunoXome™/Caelyx™
  - mitoxantrone
  - bleomycin
  - actinomycin D.
- Plant-derived drugs:
  - vinca alkaloids
- taxanes
  - docetaxel/paclitaxel
  - etoposide
  - topoisomerase I and II inhibitors
  - camptothecin/irinotecan (CPT-II)/topetecan.

ALKYLATOR AND PLATINUM DRUGS

The mechanism of action of these drugs involves the production of covalent adducts on the nitrogenous bases in DNA. This results in DNA interstrand cross-linking (so-called adduct formation). The result of this process is that DNA is unable to replicate. These agents are antiproliferative.

BCNU (carmustine) and CCNU (lomustine)

BCNU (given intravenously) and CCNU (given orally) are lipid-soluble agents. This allows them to cross the blood–brain barrier. They have activity in lymphoma, myeloma, melanoma and malignant glioma. Toxicities are myelosuppression, which can be delayed and severe, and emesis.

Busulphan

This drug is given orally and is used in high-dose chemotherapy prior to stem-cell transplantation. It is used in the treatment of haematological malignancies. Side effects include myelosuppression, which can be severe and prolonged, pulmonary fibrosis and skin pigmentation.

Treosulfan is an analogue of busulphan, given either intravenously or orally and is used in ovarian cancer. Myelosuppression is the main toxicity associated with it.

Carboplatin

This drug, a platinum analogue, produces DNA cross-links and so prevents DNA synthesis. The majority of drug is renally excreted. Dose reduction in renal impairment should be considered and renal monitoring is essential on treatment. It is indicated for use in ovarian cancer, lung cancer (small cell and non-small-cell), metastatic germ cell tumours (such as seminomas and teratomas), bladder cancer, endometrial cancer and leukaemia.

The dose of carboplatin to be administered is derived from the target plasma AUC. The Calvert formula is used to calculate the total dose required (see also Ovarian cancer: case study 1 in Chapter 5, p. 135):

$$\text{Total dose (mg)} = \text{target AUC} \times (\text{GFR} + 25)$$

AUC is the area under the plasma concentration versus time curve and GFR is glomerular filtration rate ml/min. Carboplatin should be used with caution in patients receiving nephrotoxic agents. It can cause hypersensitivity reactions with more than one course of therapy. Myelosuppression can be dose limiting and the nadir count is usually at day 14–21. There is a significant risk of thrombocytopenia. Electrolyte imbalances may occur and peripheral neuropathy, particularly in the elderly, can occur through neurotoxicity. Ototoxicity and nephrotoxicity occur much less frequently than cisplatin. Antiemetic drugs may be needed, although carboplatin is less emetogenic than cisplatin. The drug is given intravenously without the need for prehydration.

Cisplatin

This drug is given intravenously and is excreted renally. It is used widely, particularly in the treatment of upper gastrointestinal cancers, cervical, endometrial and ovarian cancers, lung cancers, bladder and testicular cancers and osteosarcomas. Myelosuppression may be moderate, as is emesis. The toxicities of cisplatin include nephrotoxicity, electrolyte disturbance (such as hyokalaemia and hypomagnesaemia) and neurotoxicity (such as a sensory peripheral neuropathy or ototoxicity).

Chlorambucil

Chlorambucil is given orally, the usual dose is 5–10 mg daily. In some cases, myelosuppression can be severe. Chlorambucil is also associated with pulmonary toxicity and the chance of secondary malignancies including acute myelogenous leukemia with long-term use. Its main indication of use is in Waldenstrom's macroglobinaemia, lymphomas (both Hodgkin's and non-Hodgkin's) and chronic lymphocytic leukaemia. It is used occasionally in the treatment of myeloma and ovarian cancer. Skin rashes can occur, with the development of Stevens–Johnson syndrome and toxic epidermal necrolysis. Sterility can occur and there is an increased risk of secondary malignancies including acute myelogenous leukaemia.

Cyclophosphamide

This alkylating agent relies on activation by the cytochrome P450 system to its active metabolites. It is well absorbed orally but can also be given intravenously. It is used in the treatment of breast cancer, bladder, chronic lymphocytic leukaemia, non-Hodgkin's lymphoma, sarcoma, ovarian cancer and neuroblastoma. It is usually used as part of combination chemotherapy. It should be used with caution in renal impairment and fluid intake should be at least 2–3 L/day to reduce the risk of haemorrhagic cystitis particularly at high doses.

There are interactions with antiepileptic drugs that induce the P450 system, such as phenytoin. There is an interaction with anticoagulants and digoxin. Other toxicities include myelosuppression, gastrointestinal toxicity, cardiotoxicity (with high doses), alopecia, secondary malignancies, immunosuppression and hypersensitivity reactions.

Cyclophosphamide produces toxic metabolites. One of these is acrolein, which is excreted in the urine and, in 10% of patients, causes haemorrhagic cystitis (severe cystitis associated with bleeding from the bladder). The principles of preventing this condition include good hydration and administration of 2-mercaptoethane or mesna, which inactivates acrolein in the urine.

The nadir blood count occurs between days 10–21 after intravenous use and myelosuppression may be severe. Very high doses given in high-dose stem-cell transplantation can cause lung and cardiotoxicity, such as pulmonary fibrosis and cardiomyopathy. There is also a risk of secondary malignancies and gonadal dysfunction. An example regimen is the CMF (cyclophosphamide methotrexate and 5-fluorouracil) regimen which is widely used in breast cancer.

Dacarbazine

This drug is used in the treatment of melanoma, sarcoma and lymphoma. It is administered intravenously. It should be used with caution in renal and hepatic impairment. Side effects include severe nausea and vomiting and myelosuppression and it is an irritant to soft tissue. A typical use of it is in the treatment of Hodgkin's lymphoma as part of the ABVD regimen (doxorubicin, bleomycin, vinblastine, dacarbazine).

Hexamethylamine

This is given orally, although absorption can be erratic. It is occasionally used in the treatment of ovarian cancer. Side effects include emesis and neurological toxicity.

Ifosfamide

This drug is usually given as a prolonged infusion. It is given with mesna and hydration to prevent haemorrhagic cystitis. It is indicated in the treatment of sarcomas, lymphoma, germ-cell malignancies and small cell lung cancer. The toxicity profile includes neurotoxicity with an impaired mental state, neuropathies and seizures. Renal and hepatotoxicity increases this possibility. A typical regimen might be ICE (ifosfamide, carboplatin and etoposide) used in lung cancer.

Mechlorethamine (nitrogen mustard)

This drug is given intravenously and has a very short half-life. It can cause severe phlebitis and sclerosis of veins. It is used in the treatment of Hodgkin's lymphoma. Typical use is in the MOPP regimen (nitrogen mustard, vincristine, procarbazine and prednisolone).

Melphalan

Melphalan can be given orally (but is subject to very variable oral bioavailability), intravenously or intraperitoneally. It has been used in the treatment of breast and ovarian cancers, lymphomas and myeloma and as high-dose therapy in haematological malignancies. Toxicity includes myelosuppression with nadir counts at 4–5 weeks after a 7-day oral course. It is also indicated for the treatment of polycythaemia rubra vera.

Mitomycin-C

This is given as part of the treatment of breast cancer and gastrointestinal malignancies, usually intravenously. In the treatment of superficial bladder cancers it is given as part of bladder instillations. Its main toxicity is delayed and prolonged myelosuppression. Nephrotoxicity and cardiomyopathy have been reported, as have respiratory complications such as pulmonary fibrosis.

Oxaliplatin

This new platinum analogue has been used in the treatment of colorectal and ovarian cancer. It is used as combination therapy with 5-fluorouracil. Its toxicity includes mild myelosuppression and peripheral neurotoxicity.

Procarbazine

This is given orally in the treatment of Hodgkin's disease and brain tumours. Side effects include myelosuppression, a hypersensitivity rash and nausea. It can interact with alcohol and cause nausea. It should be used with caution in renal impairment. A typical regimen of use is MOPP in the treatment of Hodgkin's lymphoma.

Thiotepa

This drug is usually given intravenously or intraperitoneally, especially in the palliation of ovarian cancer. It is not significantly myelosuppressive. Like most alkylators it affects reproductive organs and there is a risk of secondary malignancy such as leukaemia.

ANTIMETABOLITES

5-Fluorouracil (5-FU)

5-FU acts on both RNA and DNA synthesis and has multiple modalities of actions. It requires intracellular activation. It has poor oral absorption. In contrast to methotrexate, the addition of leucovorin increases the cellular cytotoxicity of 5-FU.

5-FU has been used to treat colorectal cancers, breast cancers, stomach and pancreatic cancers, cervical and vulval cancers, bladder cancers and head and neck tumours. It has also been used in dermatology for the treatment of actinic and solar keratoses, and superficial basal cell carcinomas (BCCs). The toxicity of 5-FU depends on how it is administered. It can be applied topically, or by bolus administration, i.v. infusion (which in some schedules can last up to 6 months) or by intra-arterial injection.

Gastrointestinal side effects include stomatitis, diarrhoea, anorexia, nausea and vomiting. Haematological toxicities include hand and foot syndrome, rashes, hyperpigmentation. Cardiac ischaemia with ST wave changes on ECG has been reported. Severe toxicities have been reported in families with a genetic deficiency of dihydropyropyrimidine dehydrogenase.

Capecitabine

Capecitabine following oral ingestion undergoes metabolic activation in the liver to be converted into 5-FU; it undergoes renal excretion.

Capecitabine is currently being used for the treatment of metastatic breast cancer resistant to anthracyclines and paclitaxel. Current schedules include a 21-day cycle with a 7-day rest period.

Important interactions include antacids and leucovorin, which increase either the plasma concentrations of capecitabine or the toxic effects of 5-FU. Patients on coumarin anticoagulants should be monitored carefully because drug levels may increase.

Common side effects of treatment are similar to those of 5-FU. Gastrointestinal side effects and myelosuppression are the most common side effects as well as the dermatological side effects of hand-and-foot syndrome.

Methotrexate

Methotrexate is an antifolate drug and is in the class of antimetabolite drugs. It acts to inhibit dihydrofolate reductase, a key enzyme in the *de novo* synthesis of nucleotide synthesis. It enters cells through a specific transport system and, intracellularly, undergoes a process called polyglutamination, which gives it a long intracellular half-life. It is distributed widely through the body and is metabolised within the liver and renally excreted. Resistance mechanisms to methotrexate action includes reduced intracellular entry and decreased polyglutamination. It is administered orally, intramuscularly or intrathecally. Its range of use extends from the treatment of solid tumours such as breast, head and neck and osteogenic sarcomas through to meningeal leukaemia and non-Hodgkin's lymphoma. Patients with choriocarcinoma and hydatidiform moles can be cured with methotrexate drug use. Combination drug use of methotrexate includes its use in breast cancer, head and neck cancers, lymphomas, osteosarcoma and lung cancers. It has also been used intrathecally in acute lymphocytic leukaemia.

Patients need to be warned not to take folate supplements unless prescribed as rescue particularly after high-dose methotrexate treatment. It should be used with caution in patients with renal impairment and the dose should be titrated with creatine clearance. Full blood count (FBC), liver function tests (LFTs) and ureas and electrolytes (U&E) should be monitored, initially weekly, when commencing methotrexate. Patients with pleural effusions and ascites may be at increased risk of methotrexate toxicity.

Drugs that interact with methotrexate include penicillins and cephalosporins, aspirin and NSAIDs, which all act to inhibit the renal excretion of methotrexate. There is an interaction with warfarin, resulting in a need to watch the International Normalised Ratio (INR) closely and omeprazole can increase serum methotrexate levels.

Toxicities of methotrexate include:

- Haematological: bone marrow suppression including anaemia, neutropenia and thrombocytopenia. This usually occurs at around day 10 after the start of treatment.
- Gastrointestinal: stomatitis or mucositis, usually around day 3–5 after treatment, diarrhoea, which if severe can lead to sepsis, and mild nausea and vomiting; portal fibrosis and cirrhosis have also been documented.
- Renal: renal toxicity requiring admission, alkalinisation of urine and hydration.
- Neurological toxicities: particularly after the use of intrathecal methotrexate, include headache, fever and meningism.
- Dermatological erythematous skin reactions have also been documented.
- Other toxicities include pneumonitis (cough and fever), photosensitivity, pruritus and menstrual irregularities.

Methotrexate: preventing deaths The National Patient Safety Agency alerted the NHS about the risks associated with the use of methotrexate. Oral methotrexate is prescribed both in primary and secondary care for the treatment of rheumatoid arthritis and severe psoriasis. There have been over 50 deaths or serious harm associated with the use of oral methotrexate over a 10-year period in England. The drug is usually prescribed as a weekly dose and errors in prescribing and packaging have been cited as reasons for these events. There has been a change in the drug formulation so that the 10 mg dose looks different to the 2.5 mg tablet.

In other medical specialties and primary care, low-dose methotrexate is also prescribed for the treatment of rheumatoid arthritis and severe psoriasis with shared care guidelines explicit between primary and secondary care. Liver toxicity, including cirrhosis, can occur with long-term low-dose use.

Gemcitabine

Gemcitabine is given intravenously and undergoes intracellular metabolic activation to metabolites, which interfere with DNA synthesis. Excretion is through the urinary tract and thus patients with renal or hepatic impairment should be monitored carefully.

Gemcitabine is currently being used for patients with locally advanced or metastatic adenocarcinoma of the pancreas. It has also been used in the treatment of breast cancer, lung cancer, bladder and head and neck cancers either as a single agent or in combination.

Current schedules include weekly administration for 7 weeks followed by 1 week's rest. Toxicities include myelosuppression, life-threatening oesophagitis or pneumonitis if there is concurrent radiotherapy, gastrointestinal and flu-like symptoms. Its advantage of use includes low myelotoxicity, low non-haematological toxicity and a favourable tolerability profile. Phase II trials in metastatic breast cancer had single-agent response rates of 25–46%. In pretreated metastatic breast cancer, gemcitabine and the taxanes produce response rates of 41–51%.

Hydroxyurea

Hydroxyurea is an example of a ribonucleotide reductase inhibitor, a key enzyme in DNA synthesis. It is available in tablet form and has a half-life of around 5 hours.

Most prescriptions in primary care are issued for the maintenance treatment of essential thrombocythaemias and polycythaemia rubra vera. In oncology it is used for the treatment of melanoma, chronic myeloid leukaemia (CML), ovarian cancers, acute leukaemia and renal cell cancers.

Capsules can be opened and added to the patient's food to allow compliance.

Leucopenia is a common side effect. Changes in the mean red cell volume have been noted. Acute leukaemia has been noted with use and long-term use may lead to gastrointestinal symptoms such as diarrhoea and constipation. Dermatological side effects include lower leg users and skin and nail hyperpigmentation.

6-MP

Mercaptopurine (6-MP) is used in the treatment of acute leukaemia. Azathioprine is metabolised to mercaptopurine and there is an interaction with allopurinol.

Ralitrexed

This drug inhibits thymidylate synthase, a key enzyme in the *de novo* synthesis of DNA. It has been given intravenously and is used in patients who have failed or cannot take fluorouracil and folinic acid. Side effects include severe diarrhoea and myelosuppression. It should be used with caution in patients with renal and hepatic impairment. Its use is much limited now.

ANTITUMOUR ANTIBIOTICS

Anthracyclines

Doxorubicin hydrochloride (Adriamycin®) This drug can exert its cytotoxic effect through free radical formation, inhibition of the enzyme topoisomerase II and DNA binding. Resistance mechanisms to anthracyclines include the expression of P-glycoprotein (P-gp), which when expressed on tumour cells leads to the efflux of cytotoxic agents from the cell. The expression of this leads to multidrug resistance (MDR). Doxorubicin is used widely in the treatment of breast cancer, lung cancer, upper gastrointestinal tumours, lymphomas and sarcoma. It is metabolised through the liver after intravenous administration and must be used with care in patients with liver disease. Toxicities include myelosuppression, alopecia and emesis; doxorubicin hydrochloride is a vesicant. Cardiotoxicity is seen with cumulative doses which exceed 450 mg/m^2.

The mechanism of cardiotoxicity is related to the production of iron-dependent free radicals, which may lead to cardiac cell membrane damage. Iron chelators such as bisdioxopiperazine may reduce this toxicity effect. Epirubicin, a synthetic analogue, has similar activity to doxorubicin with less cardiotoxicity and daunorubicin is used instead of doxorubicin for the treatment of acute non-lymphocytic leukaemia.

Liposomal drugs

DaunoXome™ This is daunorubicin encapsulated by distearoylphosphatidylcholine/cholesterol.

Caelyx™ This is polyethylene glycol (PEG)-coated liposomal encapsulation of doxorubicin. Both DaunoXome™ and Caelyx™ have fewer side effects than standard anthracyclines, although myelosuppression remains a problem. This type of drug has been used in AIDS-associated Kaposi's sarcoma.

Mitoxantrone

This is a synthetic version of the anthracyclines used in the treatment of breast cancer, combination regimens in lymphomas and in the treatment of some leukaemias. It is given intravenously. It is less cardiotoxic than standard anthracycline drugs but cardiac monitoring is necessary with cumulative doses.

Bleomycin

This is an example of an antitumour antibiotic drug. It can cause cell death by causing the death of DNA strands. The intravenous method of delivery is the most effective but bleomycin is also given into the intrapleural space as treatment for malignant pleural effusions. It is eliminated through the kidneys and patients with renal impairment are at risk of drug toxicity. Patients should have their creatine clearance checked before starting therapy, and renal function checked during courses. Interactions with other drugs such as cisplatin may worsen renal function. Bleomycin is used to treat germ cell tumours (e.g. testicular cancer), Hodgkin's and non-Hodgkin's lymphoma, head and neck cancers, cervical cancers and as a pleurodesis agent in the treatment of malignant pleural effusions and ascites.

There is an increased risk of pulmonary toxicity with cumulative dosing of bleomycin (usually > 400 units of bleomycin). The clinical signs of this include dyspnoea, cough and inspiratory crackles. Chest X-ray may show lung infiltrates and oxygen saturations may be low. Lung function tests (e.g. vital capacity) and chest X-ray should be done before starting treatment and before each cycle of treatment. High concentrations of administered oxygen, especially at the time of surgery, may worsen this toxicity. Other side effects include the possibility of anaphylaxis, fevers and chills, skin rashes including blistering and hyperpigmentation. Typical combinations of drug regimens using bleomycin include ABVD (doxorubicin, bleomycin, vinblastine, dacarbazine) used in Hodgkin's disease, BEP (bleomycin, etoposide and cisplatin) used in testicular cancer, PmitCEBO (prednisolone, mitoxantrone, cyclophosphamide, etoposide, bleomycin and vincristine) used in non-Hodgkin's lymphoma and VAPEC-B (vincristine, doxorubicin, prednisolone, etoposide, cyclophosphamide and bleomycin) used in Hodgkin's and non-Hodgkin's disease.

Actinomycin-D

This drug is given intravenously and is useful in the treatment of choriocarcinoma, Ewing's sarcoma and rhabdomyosarcoma. The toxicity profile includes gastrointestinal side effects, myelosuppression and alopecia. It is highly vesicant and can cause skin necrosis.

PLANT-DERIVED AGENTS

Vinca alkaloids

This class of drugs includes vincristine and vinblastine, which are derived from the periwinkle tree, and vindesine and vinorelbine, which are structural analogues. They all act to inhibit spindle formation at the time of mitosis (the microtubules are essential for cellular function, they maintain cell shape, mobility, adhesion and intracellular integrity) and are all drugs that exhibit MDR.

Role of vinca alkaloids

- Vinblastine: role in breast cancer, testicular and haematological cancers.
- Vincristine: also used in Wilms' tumour, Ewing's sarcoma, neuroblastoma and rhabdomyosarcoma.
- Vindesine: has similar activity to the above two drugs.
- Vinorelbine: active in non-small-cell cancer, ovarian cancer and breast cancer and Hodgkin's disease.

Toxicities:

- Neurological toxicity: vincristine and vindesine, and less so with vinorelbine.
- Haematological toxicities: vinblastine.

TAXANES

Paclitaxel (Taxol™)

This drug originates from the bark of the Pacific yew tree *Taxus brevifolia*. Its main use is in the treatment of breast and ovarian cancers. It works by disrupting normal cell division, particularly affecting mircotubular function within the cell. It is administered intravenously either as an infusion over 2–3 hours or over 24 hours. Allergic reactions following administration of the drug can lead to hypotension with acute anaphylaxis. Patients receive premedication with steroids and antihistamines, which attenuates the allergic response. Myelosuppression may be dose limiting and does occur early. Other toxicities include a sensory neuropathy, which may be reversible, arrhythmias, alopecia and flu-like symptoms.

Docetaxel (Taxotere™)

This is a semi-synthetic analogue of paclitaxel. It is usually given as a 1-hour intravenous infusion. It should be used with caution, like paclitaxel, in patients with abnormal hepatic function. Anaphylaxis rates of around 25% are similar to paclitaxel and occur at the beginning of the infusion. Premedication with steroids attenuates this response and also a capillary-leak-like syndrome characterised by oedema, effusions and weight gain. This occurs with cumulative dosing and is reversible, but can be dose limiting. Neutropenia can occur early in treatment; alopecia and a neuropathy do occur.

Etoposide

This drug is an epipodophyllotoxin analogue that affects cell division through disruption of mitosis. It is given orally and sometimes intravenously. It is excreted renally and toxicity increases in the presence of renal toxicity. Toxicities include gastrointestinal, myelosuppression and alopecia. It is used in the treatment of germ cell tumours, lung cancer (small cell), ovarian and haematological cancers.

Topoisomerase I and II inhibitors

Nuclear topoisomerase I and II are DNA enzymes that form a complex structure with supercoiled DNA that ultimately leads to DNA replication and repair. It was found that topoisomerase I levels can be higher in tumour cells and thus this compound became an interesting target for chemotherapy.

Camptothecin/Irinotecan (CPT-II)/Topetecan

Camptothecin and its analogues irinotecan (CPT-II) and topetecan block DNA repair through their action on topoisomerase I.

Topetecan is usually given as an intravenous bolus every 3 weeks. It is associated with myelosuppression, alopecia and emesis. It is used in the treatment of breast cancer, relapsed ovarian cancer, lung cancer and head and neck cancers.

Irinotecan or CPT-II is given intravenously every 3 or 4 weeks. It is given for relapsed colorectal cancer after 5-FU treatment, lung cancer and ovarian cancer. It is associated with severe myelosuppression. Other toxicities include sever diarrhoea, which may cause dehydration and can present within 24 hours of treatment or late in treatment; it can be treated by an anticholinergic.

References

ATAC Trialists Group 2002 Anastrozole alone or in combination with tamoxifen versus tamoxifen alone for adjuvant treatment of postmenopausal women with early breast cancer: first results of the ATAC randomised trial. The Lancet 359:2131–2139

Drugs and Therapeutics Bulletin (DTB) 2003 Should aromatase inhibitors replace tamoxifen? DTB 41:57–58

Mouridsen H et al 2003 Phase III study of letrozole versus tamoxifen as first line therapy of advanced breast cancer in postmenopausal women: analysis of survival and update of efficacy from the Letrozole Breast Cancer Group. Journal of Clinical Oncology 21:2101–2109

Ravdin S 2002 Aromatase inhibitors for the endocrine adjuvant treatment of breast cancer. The Lancet 359:2126–2127

Rutz HP 2002 Effect of corticosteroid use on treatment of solid tumours. The Lancet 360:1969–1970

Useful websites

www.cancerbackup.org.uk
www.cancersourcemd.com

CHAPTER 4

Complications of cancer chemotherapy

Chapter contents

INTRODUCTION

The ideal cancer drug is one that is selective for the target cancer so that it can exert its anticancer effect without compromising normal tissue and causing host toxicity. The reality is that all cytotoxic drugs will have some degree of toxicity because of their antiproliferative effect. Normal cells require normal functioning of DNA and RNA synthesis. These are the targets of anticancer drugs and thus cells in bone marrow and gastrointestinal tracts, which have cells with a fast turnover, are also affected. Future drug development is going to be dependent on new drugs with greater selectivity through an understanding of molecular biology and computer technology.

The success of cytotoxic chemotherapy is related to the supportive care that is now possible. For example:

- The use of high-dose steroids such as dexamethasone and 5-hydroxytryptamine antagonists (e.g. ondansetron) as antiemetics.
- Colony stimulating factors, e.g. G-CSF and GM-CSF.
- The use of prophylactic antifungal and antibacterial agents, and the aggressive treatment of viral, fungal and bacterial infection: immunosuppression should be monitored vigilantly for potential infective complications, particularly in the presence of a neutropenia.
- Analgesic drugs: cancers can be painful and cancer chemotherapy is used to palliate. The use of opiates is common in the management of the cancer patients and allows patients to progress through courses of treatment.
- Bisphosphonate treatment in patients with osteolytic bone metastases to help bone healing and reduce pain.

In the future it is possible that pharmacogenetics will help predict which patients are at more risk of suffering complications. For example, it is known dihydropyrimidine dehydrogenase (DHD) is the rate-limiting enzyme in the metabolism of 5-FU. Studies have looked at the relationship between variations in the gene that encodes DHD and lack of DHD activity, which in turn is associated with severe toxicity in patients who are given 5-FU chemotherapy.

The development of new therapies, particularly new targeted therapies in combination with standard cytotoxic agents, may lead to different and novel toxicity profiles. Clinical studies will need to identify these side effects and methods developed to optimise supportive care. It is clear that many drugs cause multiple side effects and the principle of management must be to maintain vigilance for predictable complications.

ECOG COMMON TOXICITY CRITERIA

The ECOG common toxicity criteria (CTC) are used to assess the response to treatment in terms of the toxicity that patients may experience after chemotherapy or radiotherapy. These cover haematological, renal, gastrointestinal, liver, pulmonary, cardiac, dermatological and neurological toxicity, as well as metabolic side effects. Grade 0 refers to no toxicity whereas grade 4 reflects the most severe toxicity (Table 4.1) (the guidelines are available online at: www.ecog.org/general/ctc.pdf and see also Appendix 2).

TABLE 4.1 Example of ECOG common toxicity criteria for vomiting

Grade	0	1	2	3	4
Toxicity	None	1 episode in 24 hours	2–5 episodes in 24 hours	6–10 episodes in 24 hours	> 10 episodes in 24 hours requiring parenteral support

HAEMATOLOGICAL COMPLICATIONS

The acute effect of chemotherapy-induced damage to the bone marrow is toxicity to the stem cells that are the precursors of peripheral blood components. Granulocytes have a half-life of 6 hours, platelets 10 days and erythrocytes 120 days. Therefore the most common impairment of bone marrow function leads to a leucopenia and a transient thrombocytopenia. People at risk of haematological toxicity include those who have already received chemotherapy and those with bone marrow involvement due to disease. The rate of clearance of drug and active metabolites also has a major influence on potential toxicity, as does the type of drug (e.g. antimetabolites versus non-cycle-dependent chemotherapeutic agents) and the schedule of the drug. Pharmacogenetics is an important factor to consider (i.e. gene allelic variations that might predispose to toxicity). The knowledge of how a drug is metabolised and which pathways are activated can be used to modulate the action of a drug. For example, the action of methotrexate is to inhibit folate metabolism and thus a means of rescuing the patient after methotrexate administration is to use leucovorin, which provides folates, within 48 hours of drug administration.

In patients with chronic bone marrow damage (e.g. showing leucopenia) dose reductions of chemotherapy agents may need to be given. These patients may also be at risk of myelodysplastic syndromes and secondary leukaemias. The alkylating agents in particular are responsible for late complications.

It is important to monitor for nadirs of white cell counts and platelets after chemotherapy administration. As bone marrow cells are dividing cells they are most sensitive to the antiproliferative effects of chemotherapy. As chemotherapy is administered, the circulating supply of dividing marrow cells reduces and the blood counts fall to a low point, the nadir. One of the reasons why chemotherapy is administered on a monthly basis is to allow the bone marrow to recover through increased stem cell production. Depending on the regimen and the drug used, there is some variation in the nadir time but 10 days after chemotherapy administration is quite common.

ANAEMIA

The effect of bone marrow suppression is to cause anaemia with the patient reporting dyspnoea, light-headedness and lethargy. Human recombinant formulations of erythropoietin – epoetin-α and epoetin-β – are licensed for the treatment of anaemia in adults who receive chemotherapy. Epoetin-β is also licensed in the prevention of anaemia in adults with solid tumours treated with platinum agents. Randomised trials have shown that administration of these subcutaneous compounds reduces the need for blood transfusion, increases haemoglobin levels and improves quality of life. They are indicated for use in patients with solid or non-myeloid tumours with haemoglobin levels below 10 g/dL. Side effects of treatment include a rise in blood pressure and in platelet counts; these need to be monitored during treatment. In prolonged use, red cell aplasia has been reported and in this situation the drug should be discontinued. Blood transfusions may be indicated particularly if the Hb is < 8 g/dL. Autoimmune haemolytic anaemias can also occur as a side effect of the drug administered, and this applies especially for the platinum agents. The haemolytic–uraemic syndrome has been associated with mitomycin-C as well as the platinum agents.

LEUCOPENIA AND NEUTROPENIA

The development of leucopenia and neutropenia can put patients at risk of opportunistic infection. Risk factors for febrile neutropenia in patients receiving chemotherapy include bone marrow involvement, prior myelosuppressive therapy and concomitant or prior radiation therapy. The importance of preventive measures, such as good hygiene and avoiding exposure to people with known infections, are important. These patients are at risk of febrile neutropenic sepsis, an oncological emergency necessitating rehydration, intravenous antibiotics and intensive support. In severe neutropenia there might be a need for growth factors such as G-CSF. All cancer units will have guidelines on the treatment of febrile neutropenia, which will include which antibiotics to use and when to initiate G-CSF. If a patient is undergoing high-dose chemotherapy then the use of G-CSF is usually incorporated as part of the chemotherapy regimen. However, with conventional chemotherapy the use of G-CSF is usually reserved for when there is a febrile neutropenia that has not responded to antibiotics, antifungals and the absolute neutrophil count is below 0.5×10^9/L for more than 10 days (Dearnley 2002). The importance of the absolute neutrophil nadir count after the first chemotherapy dose is that it can be used as a predictor of subsequent neutropenic events and thus dose reduction may be needed.

THROMBOCYTOPENIA

A low number of platelets means there is a need to avoid trauma, to ensure that no i.m. injections are given and that signs of bleeding, such as melaena, petechiae and haematuria, are monitored. Alcohol and drugs such as aspirin, which may worsen bleeding tendency, should be avoided. Platelet transfusions are used for severe thrombocytopenias.

Typical drugs causing myelosuppression include the:

- Antimetabolites: 5-FU, methotrexate and cytosine. For methotrexate in particular it is important to reduce dose in renal impairment, to drain any pleural effusion or ascites and to use folinic acid rescue after high doses.
- Alkylating drugs: chlorambucil, cyclophosphamide, ifosfamide, melphalan and mustine.
- Antibiotic drugs: bleomycin and mitomycin-C.
- Anthracyclines: daunorubicin, doxorubicin, epirubicin, idarubicin and the anthracenedione mitozantrone.
- Platinum agents: carboplatin and cisplatin, where renal function is important and dose should be reduced in renal impairment.
- The vinca alkaloids: vinblastine, vincristine and vindesine.
- Miscellaneous drugs: including dacarbazine, etoposide and procarbazine.

GASTROINTESTINAL TOXICITY

Common side effects after chemotherapy include nausea and vomiting, diarrhoea and constipation and oral mucositis. This may lead onto dehydration, weight loss, and electrolyte disturbances such as hyponatraemia.

The mechanism of emesis involves stimulation of neuroreceptors in the central nervous system, particularly in the chemoreceptor trigger zone in the medulla. Dopamine receptors, serotonin and acetylcholine neurotransmitters act on this area and hence the role of antiemetics is to inhibit or block the action of these neurotransmitters.

Emesis may occur during chemotherapy treatment or it may be delayed and occur after chemotherapy has been administered; 25% of patients have what is called anticipatory emesis, which occurs before chemotherapy is administered and is a response to the anticipation of receiving chemotherapy. It mainly occurs in patients who perhaps have not received adequate antiemesis in previous courses of treatment. Other reasons as to why patients develop nausea and vomiting must also be considered, such as bowel obstruction.

Most patients receive antiemetics before their chemotherapy but recurrent and delayed symptoms require further antiemetic use. Many cytotoxic agents are known to cause emesis and in combination therapy the drug with the most emetogenic potential should be identified to provide adequate control of symptoms. Examples of cytotoxic drugs with emetogenic potential are given below (Gralla 1999):

- Severely emetogenic drugs: cisplatin, dacarbazine and mechlorethamine.

- Moderately emetogenic drugs: carboplatin, cyclophosphamide, cytarabine, mitoxantrone and oxaliplatin.
- Low emetogenic drugs: docetaxel, 5-FU, gemcitabine and paclitaxel.
- Drugs that are least likely to cause emesis: bleomycin, chlorambucil, low-dose methotrexate, melphalan and vincristine.

The range of antiemetics is wide and it may be necessary to experiment with differing agents until the symptoms resolve. Evidence-based guidelines are available as to which antiemetics to use (Gralla 1999). Phenothiazines such as prochlorperazine, metoclopramide, dexamethasone, and 5-HT$_3$ antagonists such as ondansetron and granistron are typical antiemetic drugs used to combat this side effect. Other drugs used include haloperidol, benzodiazepines and semisynthetic cannabinoids such as nabilone.

Thus antiemetics can be tailored to the treatment and used both in the setting of acute onset and delayed onset nausea and vomiting. Example regimens used for the different range of emetogenic drugs are given below in the setting of acute onset nausea and vomiting during treatment:

- Severely emetogenic regimens, such as a cisplatin-containing regimen: use a 5-HT$_3$ drug such as ondansetron in combination with a steroid such as dexamethasone. The same regimen would be used in a regimen with moderate emetogenic potential, such as when using carboplatin.
- Regimens with a low emetogenic potential could use a single antiemetic agent.

In delayed-onset nausea and vomiting, combinations of steroid, e.g. oral dexamethasone with metoclopramide, have been shown to be better than oral steroids on their own. Single 5-HT$_3$ agents are used for regimens that are moderately to severely emetogenic in the delayed setting. Drugs that could be prescribed in the community for delayed-onset nausea or vomiting include phenothiazines, metoclopramide, domperidone and haloperidol. Different routes of administration could include subcutaneous injection or rectal administration.

Single and drug combinations may cause a variety of side effects, as illustrated by the use of 5-FU chemotherapy and methotrexate (Table 4.2), and different modalities of supportive care will need to be given with vigilance that other comorbidity may influence care.

ORAL COMPLICATIONS

Oral complications of cancer chemotherapy can lead to pain with reduced oral intake and resulting weight loss. An example of such toxicity is mucositis; the drugs that have been shown to particularly cause this include the antimetabolites such as 5-FU and methotrexate, doxorubicin, bleomycin and busulphan. The possible effects include treatment delays and dose

TABLE 4.2 Side effects of chemotherapy with 5-FU and methotrexate (from Gralla et al 1999)

Drug	Side effect/toxicity	Treatment
5-FU	GI: stomatitis and diarrhoea	Mouth washes/dietary advice Antidiarrhoeal agents Watch for signs of dehydration Supportive care and monitoring for anaemia, leucopenia and thrombocytopenia
Methotrexate	GI: stomatitis and diarrhoea Renal impairment (high-dose) Liver fibrosis (low-dose, chronic)	As above Admit for rehydration Monitor LFTs for rises in transaminases Supportive care and monitoring for anaemia, leucopenia and thrombocytopenia needed. Patients need good support during this difficult period of chemotherapy administration and behavioural and psychological support may need to be available

GI, gastrointestinal; LFT, liver function test.

reductions with possible effect on outcome and survival (Mead 2002). Mucositis can be a dose-limiting toxic effect and is influenced by the scheduling of the drugs. The presence of mucositis can lead to mouth ulceration with the possibility of sepsis because of microorganisms taking advantage of weak mucosal barriers to infection. It is important to recognise that infection may be caused by bacterial, fungal or viral infection. For example, oral candidiasis can lead to systemic candidal infection. Similarly, infection with viruses such as herpes and cytomegalovirus are important to identify and treat promptly to prevent systemic disease in an immune compromised patient.

Good oral care with mouth rinsing and regular teeth brushing is an important preventive measure. Sucking ice during treatment reduces the oral mucosa to drug exposure and may reduce the chances of mucositis (Mead 2002). Other measures include the use of antacids, topical anaesthetics and antihistamines. Nutritional advice is important during this phase of treatment and nutritional supplements may be needed. In some cases, the level of mucositis is such that a nasogastric tube may be necessary.

Other oral complications include dental pulp infections and periodontal infections.

DIARRHOEA

Diarrhoea is a common symptom after chemotherapy administration, particularly after the use of antimetabolites such as methotrexate, 5-FU and capecitabine, and the platinum agent cisplatin. Standard antidiarrhoeal agents are used to treat diarrhoea, along with dehydration formulas, although admission for intravenous fluid replacement might be necessary. The vinca alkaloid group of drugs, such as vincristine, are particularly liable to cause constipation. Stimulants such as senokot and osmotic laxatives such as lactulose can help, along with dietary advice and good fluid intake.

HEPATOTOXICITY

Hepatic toxicity can vary from mild rises in transaminases to hepatic necrosis. Pre-existing liver disease and hepatic metastases will have an effect on hepatic function and the response of the liver to chemotherapy drugs. Thus, selecting a suitable chemotherapy agent and modifying the dose administered in the presence of coexisting hepatic disease and comorbidity is important. Following treatment, abnormalities of liver function tests (LFTs) may be due to the effects of chemotherapy rather than to progressive disease, and this is important in deciding on the next dose of chemotherapy to be administered. Complications of chemotherapy treatment, such as immune suppression, lead to the possibility of acute hepatitis due, for example, to viral infections and these must be borne in mind when abnormal LFTs are noted. Most hepatotoxic drug reactions are idiosyncratic immunological reactions and are not dose dependent (King & Perry 2001).

Examples of hepatic complications related to drug administration include fibrosis and cirrhosis associated with antimetabolites, and to methotrexate in particular. Methotrexate used for maintenance therapy in children with acute leukaemia has been associated with hepatic cirrhosis and fibrosis. Low-dose methotrexate administered over a long period for chronic conditions such as rheumatoid arthritis and psoriasis has been implicated in the development of fibrosis and cirrhosis.

Fatty change, cholestasis and hepatic necrosis may be the sequelae of drug administration and dose modifications might be necessary. A large number of chemotherapy drugs can be implicated in some degree of hepatic toxicity, including drugs from the alkylating agents, nitrosurea and antitumour antibiotic and platinum agents.

RENAL COMPLICATIONS

The renal complications of cancer treatment can originate either from the direct nephrotoxicity of the drug on the kidneys or from the effect of the interaction between the anticancer drug and the effect on the cancer, which can result in a metabolic state that could harm the renal structures. The renal complication of treatment may occur early (e.g. during the first course of treatment), during cumulative dosing or as a late complication after treatment has been completed. The following drugs are highly nephrotoxic: the platinum agent cisplatin, the antifolate methotrexate and, in high doses, mithramycin and mitomycin. When administering these drugs it is important to monitor renal function because patients can be asymptomatic but with ongoing renal damage. Knowledge of the pharmacokinetics of a drug is important. Drugs may produce toxic metabolites and these, not the parent drug, might cause damage. Different treatment modalities might also have a high risk of renal toxicity, such as when patients with haematological malignancies receive autologous peripheral blood stem-cell transplantation. Examples of nephrotoxicity include:

- tumour lysis syndrome
- urate nephropathy
- tubular abnormalities
- glomerular dysfunction.

Tumour lysis syndrome is an oncological emergency. It occurs after the administration of anticancer drugs that lead to cell death in chemosensitive tumours, such as lymphomas and leukaemias, but it can also occur in the treatment of testicular cancer. The leakage of electrolytes from dying cells leads to hyperkalaemia, hyperphosphataemia, hypocalcaemia and hyperuricaemia. Acute renal failure may be precipitated by the depositions of uric acid and calcium phosphate crystals in the renal tubules. There is the risk of arrhythmias and sudden death in these patients. Patients who may be at risk include those with extensive and aggressive tumours, pre-existing renal disease and a high lactate dehydrogenase. Patients should be well hydrated before treatment. Prophylactic allopurinol is given and urinary alkalinisation is necessary to maintain a neutral pH to prevent or treat this syndrome. Some patients might need haemodialysis.

Cisplatin can cause both acute and chronic renal failure, predominately due to tubular damage, which in turn can cause not only decreases in glomerular filtration rate (GFR) but also severe electrolyte disturbances, such as hypomagnesaemia and hypocalcaemia, and loss of sodium in the urine leading to postural hypotension. The important management principle is to prehydrate patients before treatment, to ensure that patients with compromised renal function do not receive cisplatin and either to withdraw the drug when toxicity is recognised or to reduce the dose and monitor and treat the electrolyte disturbances (Patterson & Reams 2002). Other drugs with which particular care needs to be taken include ifosfamide and cyclophosphamide. Ifosfamide causes a haemorrhagic cystitis as well as a proximal tubular defect, whereas cyclophosphamide causes haemorrhagic cystitis and the syndrome of inappropriate ADH secretion, which is associated with hyponatraemia. Methotrexate is important because at high doses it may precipitate within the tubules, leading to higher serum levels and the possibility of bone marrow suppression. Streptozocin is associated with a tubular defect, as are lomustine and carmustine. Mitomycin-C chemotherapy can cause a haemolytic anaemic syndrome with renal failure; this occurs with cumulative dosing. Combinations of drugs, such as cisplatin and methotrexate, may potentiate the possibility of renal toxicity.

PULMONARY COMPLICATIONS

PULMONARY INFECTION

After cancer chemotherapy, patients are at risk of myelosuppression and immunosuppression. This opens up the risk of opportunistic infections. The type of infection is dependent on the degree and type of immunological and myelosuppression (Table 4.3). The underlying malignancy also makes a difference, so that those patients with pulmonary lesions may be more liable to develop infections from organisms that normally colonise the oropharynx and upper airways.

When faced with a patient who has received chemotherapy recently, the GP or primary care healthcare professional must be aware of the potential for

TABLE 4.3   Immunological deficits and types of infections (adapted from Rolston 2001)

Type of deficit	Type of infections
Neutropenia	Gram-negative infections, e.g. *Escherichia coli*, *Pseudomonas aeruginosa* Gram-positive cocci, e.g. *Staphylococcus aureus*, *Streptococcus viridans* Fungal infections, e.g. *Aspergillus* spp. (usually in severe and prolonged neutropenia)
Impaired cellular immunity	Viral infections, e.g. cytomegalovirus, herpes viruses Bacterial infections, e.g. *Legionella* spp., *Mycobacterium* spp. Fungal, e.g. *Aspergillus* spp., *Candida* spp. Protozoan, e.g. *Pneumocystis carinii* infection
Impaired humoral immunity	Infections with *Streptococcus pneumoniae*, *Haemophilus influenzae*

infection in the neutropenic patient. The nadir white cell count may not be for up to 10 days after chemotherapy and the response to infection may be blunted. Symptoms and signs of infection may be atypical and minimal because of the blunted inflammatory response; patients on steroids are a classic example of this. Vital signs such as pulse, temperature and blood pressure must be checked and, if there is any doubt, patients should be referred to secondary care. Neutropenic sepsis is an oncological emergency.

PULMONARY FIBROSIS

Chemotherapy is associated with pulmonary inflammation and fibrosis, which could lead to acute and/or chronic respiratory failure. Typical drugs that might cause pulmonary fibrosis include:

- The antimetabolite methotrexate: can cause an interstitial fibrosis with bibasilar infiltrates.
- The alkylating agents chlorambucil, cyclophosphamide and mustine.
- The antibiotic bleomycin: in this case the fibrosis is progressive. Pulmonary function and chest X-ray monitoring are important. Endothelial damage of the lung vasculature occurs. This is thought to be due to bleomycin-induced cytokines and free radicals leading to fibrosis. Men treated with bleomycin for testicular cancer are at risk of lung toxicity and a small proportion can develop a fatal pneumonitis.
- Miscellaneous: include procarbazine, mitomycin and busulphan.

Patients may present with breathlessness, fever and an acute pneumonitis. They might present acutely during chemotherapy regimens, in which setting the drug must be stopped. The syndrome may actually occur many months after chemotherapy has been completed. Treatment in the case of fibrosis is supportive. Corticosteroids are sometimes used but with varying success, depending on the causative drug.

NEUROTOXICITY

NEUROPATHIES AND CANCER CHEMOTHERAPY

Neurons and Schwann cells are slowly dividing cells and yet peripheral neurotoxicity is a significant dose-limiting side effect of many chemotherapy agents. Mechanisms of damage for some drugs remain unknown. Disturbances in microtubule structure with axonal injury have been discovered for drugs including paclitaxel and vinca alkaloids (vincristine, vinblastine and vindesine).

The platinum analogues cisplatin and oxaliplatin have neuropathy as a significant side effect, and this can be a dose-limiting toxicity (Windebank 1999). Preclinical studies have shown that cisplatin may induce apoptosis of the dorsal root ganglion neurons. Carboplatin has a less toxic side effect profile than cisplatin. The taxanes produce a distal sensory neuropathy with some recovery after completion of treatment. Combinations of taxanes and platinum agents have not produced more severe neuropathy than single-agent administration. Suramin, a drug used in hormone-refractory prostate cancer, leads to an axonal neuropathy and a severe polyradiculopathy. New agents are being developed that work to combat these side effects, including agents that augment the response of neurons to trophic agents.

CARDIAC TOXICITY

ANTHRACYCLINE USE AND CARDIAC COMPLICATIONS

Although many drugs can induce cardiac complications, the group that does this most commonly is the anthracyclines (Nelson et al 2001). Patients may develop dose-limiting cardiac toxicity, which may include supraventricular arrhythmias, dyspnoea, hypotension, pericardial effusions, congestive heart failure and acute or chronic cardiomyopathy. The onset of cardiotoxicity can be acute, subacute, chronic (high cumulative doses) or a late complication (years after completion of treatment). The normal mechanisms that protect a cell from free radicals are lacking in myocardial tissue. Anthracycline-associated cardiotoxicity is linked to the production of free radicals, which are toxic to myocardial tissue. The dose administered is particularly important and cumulative doses increase the likelihood of damage. Dose scheduling also appears to be important in that continuous dose infusion at low doses appears less toxic than large doses every 3 weeks. Risk factors associated with an increase in cardiotoxicity include previous anthracycline therapy, irradiation to the chest wall, pre-existing cardiac disease and administration with other chemotherapy drugs, such as cyclophosphamide and the taxanes. Monitoring of left ventricular ejection function, usually through multiple-gated acquisition (MUGA) scans is mandatory. Monitoring cumulative disease is all important. Analogues of daunorubicin and doxorubicin, i.e. mitoxantrone, idarubicin and epirubicin, have been developed to lessen cardiotoxicity. The same principles of watching cumulative doses apply for these drugs. The development of cardioprotective agents such as dexrazoxane and amifostine may offer cellular protection to the myocardium. Phase II studies of dexrazoxane (which acts as an iron chelator) have been encouraging in reducing the incidence of cardiotoxicity when given with an anthracycline. Preclinical trials with amifostine have been encouraging.

LATE COMPLICATIONS

A significant proportion of children who have had cancer in childhood are now surviving into adulthood. These children may well have survived treatment regimens for lymphomas and leukaemias. Currently, the average GP will have three childhood survivors on his or her register but, with advances in treatment, this figure is likely to rise (Oeffinger 2000). Surveillance and increased vigilance for the health care of these patients remains important. Health-related problems can originate from the effects of treatment. These include the risk of secondary malignancy. The risk of secondary malignancies following treatment for paediatric cancer is about 2.5–3.5%. In children who were treated for Hodgkin's disease the cumulative risk for the development of breast cancer by the age of 40 years may be as high as 35%. Late complications as a result of anthracycline chemotherapy include left ventricular dysfunction leading to congestive heart failure, particularly precipitated by pregnancy. Other late effects include pulmonary fibrosis from treatment with bleomycin or busulphan, inner ear hearing loss from cisplatin treatment, primary infertility, transfusion-related hepatitis B and C, nephrotoxicity from the use of cisplatin and unresolved psychological issues. Follow-up programmes of childhood cancer survivors are particularly important so that relapses are picked up early and treatment complications are recognised; it is also important that new cancer treatments avoid secondary long-term toxicity (Lackner 2002).

Myelodysplastic syndromes and acute myeloid leukaemia can arise as a late complication of chemotherapy. Drugs that are associated include cyclophosphamide, methotrexate, fluorouracil and anthracyclines. Alkylating agents are associated with leukaemias that develop 5–7 years after treatment, whereas anthracyclines can give rise to secondary leukaemias 6 months to 5 years after treatment.

Tamoxifen is associated with an increase in the risk of endometrial cancer because of its progestogenic effect on the endometrium. This is more likely to develop with women who take tamoxifen for more than 5 years.

Women treated with chemotherapy agents such as alkylating agents are more liable to develop amenorrhoea, premature menopause and menopausal symptoms, which may be more severe than the normal biochemical changes of a natural menopause. Drugs liable to do this include tamoxifen, cyclophosphamide, methotrexate and doxorubicin. Tamoxifen can cause symptoms of the menopause. Women who have been treated for breast cancer are advised to wait for 2 years before becoming pregnant, not because of possible teratogenic effects of previous chemotherapy but because of the risk of recurrence. In those women who do become pregnant after treatment there has not been shown to be a higher incidence of congenital anomalies or abortion. It is not known what the risk of recurrence of breast cancer is in women who have had treatment who need in vitro fertilisation to overcome infertility (Radford 1999).

Bone mineral density diminishes with amenorrhoea caused by chemotherapy. The loss is similar to what happens during the natural menopause. The strategies used to prevent bone mineral loss include the use of bisphosphonates, smoking cessation, exercise, a good intake of calcium and treatment of metabolic or endocrine disorders.

Men treated in childhood with chemotherapy before puberty can develop gonadal dysfunction. Chemotherapy used for the treatment of Hodgkin's lymphoma can have a profound effect on male spermatogenesis. Alkylating drugs in particular can cause low sperm counts and the chemotherapy regimens used in the treatment of Hodgkin's lymphoma (MOPP), cancer of the testis (cisplatin, bleomycin and vinblastine; 20% of patients develop irreversible azoospermia) and sarcoma (cyclophosphamide and doxorubicin) are particularly implicated.

The news of a successful transplantation of cryopreserved autologous ovarian tissue in a previously oophorectomised woman with non-malignant disease offers hope to women who have treatment-induced sterility for cancer. However, a great deal of research is needed and many ethical considerations need to be overcome before the technique becomes standard practice.

HYPERSENSITIVITY TO CHEMOTHERAPY

Type I anaphylactic reactions to chemotherapy agents do occur; this applies to Taxol®, Taxotere®, etoposide and bleomycin. Before giving Taxol® and Taxotere®, premedication with steroids and antihistamines helps to reduce the frequency of allergic reaction. With Taxol® and Taxotere®, immediate reactions include wheeze, dyspnoea, pruritus and hypotension. Stopping the drug and treatment with fluids, steroids and an antihistamine is usually enough to resolve symptoms. Both drugs could be given again, but at a slower rate, although for some patients who react against it, this side effect may be dose limiting. Similar reactions are seen with etoposide and bleomycin. For the latter drug a test dose is usually given before the first dose.

DERMATOLOGICAL REACTIONS TO CHEMOTHERAPY

Antimetabolites, 5-FU and capecitabine can cause palmar–plantar syndrome, which results in painful erythema, pruritus and open fissuring of the skin of the hands and soles of feet. Treatment includes emollients and steroid ointments. Skin pigmentation can be caused by bleomycin, 5-FU and doxorubicin.

Alopecia may be caused in particular by the anthracyclines, antibiotics, alkylating agents, vinca alkaloids and etoposide. Alopecia can occur within a week of starting chemotherapy and is obvious by 1 month. Scalp cooling has been used in selected cases to prevent this.

Pain, swelling and erythema around an injection site may represent a mild local irritant effect of chemotherapy due to drugs such as carboplatin, docetaxel or etoposide. Drugs that cause tissue necrosis due to extravasations of drug need to be handled with extreme care. These include the anthracyclines, the vinca alkaloids and the nitrogen mustards. Drugs that are highly vesicant include epirubicin, mitomycin-C and paclitaxel, which can cause necrosis of the skin around the injection site with possible neurovascular damage. Debridement and skin grafting might be necessary in these patients. Management of the extravasation depends on the chemotherapy agent used and there should be clear guidelines within cancer units in the management of this condition.

GENITOURINARY COMPLICATIONS

Cystitis (in 10% of patients on low-dose chronic treatment) and, more rarely, haemorrhagic cystitis may occur after administration with cyclophosphamide and ifosfamide. The importance of good hydration and frequent voiding cannot be overstated here as the toxic metabolites are excreted renally. A uroprotectant drug called mesna is used during ifosfamide treatment and usually mitigates against the risk of haemorrhagic cystitis.

CANCER CHEMOTHERAPY: COMPLICATIONS IN THE OLDER PATIENT

All the pharmacokinetic processes that are necessary for effective drug delivery are affected as age increases. Thus, decreased drug absorption (important for oral drugs such as capecitabine), reduced volume of distribution, reduced hepatic drug metabolism and reduced renal function (important for drugs such as methotrexate and platinum agents) are important considerations. After the age of 70 there is a greater incidence of grade 3 and 4 myelotoxicity with chemotherapy. The incidence of gastrointestinal, CNS and cardiotoxicity all increase after the age of 65 years and cognitive impairment in particular may increase after chemotherapy administration. Factors that should be taken into account are included on many assessment scales relevant to the elderly. These include performance status, comorbidity (such as ischaemic heart disease), depression status, nutritional status and socioeconomic status. The prognosis after the cancer has been identified is important, but chemotherapy can be used to palliate.

References

Dearnley D et al 2002 Handbook of adult cancer chemotherapy schedules. The Royal Marsden NHS Trust, Surrey

Gralla RJ et al 1999 Recommendations for the use of antiemetics: evidence-based, clinical practice guidelines. American Society of Clinical Oncology. Journal of Clinical Oncology 9:2971–2994

King PD, Perry MC 2001 Hepatotoxicity of chemotherapy. The Oncologist 6(2):162–176

Lackner H 2002 Secondary effects of cancer treatment – a paediatric perspective. The Lancet Oncology 13:576–577

Mead G 2002 Management of oral mucositis associated with cancer chemotherapy. The Lancet 359:9309

Nelson MA et al 2001 Cardiovascular considerations with anthracycline use in patients with cancer. Heart Disease 3:157–168

Oeffinger KC 2000 Childhood cancer survivors and primary care physicians. Journal of Family Practitioners 49:689–690

Patterson WP, Reams GP 2002 Renal and electrolyte abnormalities due to chemotherapy. In: Perry MC (ed) The chemotherapy source book. Lippincott, Williams and Wilkins, Philadelphia

Radford J et al 1999 Fertility after treatment for cancer. British Medical Journal 319:935

Rolston KVI 2001 The spectrum of pulmonary infections in cancer patients. Current Opinion in Oncology 13(4):218–223

Windebank AJ 1999 Chemotherapeutic neuropathy. Current Opinion in Neurology 12:565–571

Useful websites

www.ecog.org/general/ctc.pdf
www.moffitt.usf.edu/pubs

CHAPTER 5

Anticancer drugs and tumour-specific disease

Chapter contents

INTRODUCTION

The aim of this chapter is to highlight anticancer drug use in the more common cancers. Examples of case management will be given, as well as some references to trials and journal papers that might be of interest. The leukaemias are outside the scope of this book.

BLADDER CANCER

There are over 5000 deaths from bladder cancer each year in the UK. Smoking and exposure to industrial aromatic amines, particularly in the dye and rubber industries, remain strong risk factors. Transitional cell carcinomas are the most common histological pattern of bladder cancers. The TNM (tumour, node, metastasis) system (Table 5.1) defines the clinical staging of bladder cancers but pathological staging is the most important prognostic factor. Grade 1 lesions are well differentiated whereas grade 3 tumours are poorly differentiated. Some have advocated that the current TNM staging system is not powerful enough to predict outcome in patients with bladder cancer. Genetic mutations in p53 and alterations in the retinoblastoma gene product pRB occur in up to 40% of bladder cancers and are poor prognostic factors.

Over 80% of patients have superficial bladder cancer. Superficial bladder cancer is defined as Tis (carcinoma in situ), Ta (non-invasive papillary cancer) or T1 (tumour invades subepithelial connective tissue) (Fig. 5.1). The muscle invasive group classed as T2–T4 has a poor prognosis of around 50% for 5-year survival.

In superficial disease, endoscopic resection and follow-up surveillance gives a 5-year survival of over 90%, although recurrences are common, with

TABLE 5.1 The TNM staging for bladder cancer

Grade	Description
Tumour (T)	
Tis	Carcinoma in situ: flat tumour confined to mucosa
TA	Non-invasive papillary cancer limited to mucosa
T1	Invades lamina propria, into connective tissue
T2a	Superficial, less than halfway muscle invasion
T2b	Deep: more than halfway muscle invasion
T3	Perivesical fat invaded (T3a microscopic, T3b macroscopic)
T4a	Invades prostate, uterus or vagina
T4b	Invades pelvic wall or abdominal wall
Lymph nodes (N)	
N0	No regional node involvement
N1	Single node, < 2 cm in largest diameter
N2	Single node 2–5 cm or multiple nodes < 5 cm
N3	Nodal involvement > 5 cm

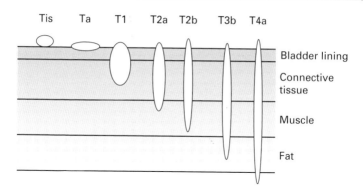

Fig. 5.1 Bladder cancer spread.

50% recurring within the first year. Carcinoma in situ (Tis) patients should be considered for intravesical therapy, as should patients with T1 tumours. This is used either to treat tumours such as carcinoma in situ, which cannot be resected, or used as adjuvant treatment after transurethral resection. Chemotherapy agents used include mitomycin-C, doxorubicin and epirubicin. Randomised trials have helped to define how long, how often and how soon these drugs are given. Adjuvant therapy may prolong the disease-free interval but does not seem to improve survival. The use of mitomycin-C is common and weekly for 6 weeks remains a popular regimen.

Intravesical therapy is recommended for recurrent disease, high-grade disease or extravesical involvement but is most effective for superficial bladder cancer. Bacille Calmette–Guérin (BCG) is particularly useful in superficial high-grade tumours (Alexandroff et al 1999). Common side effects include dysuria, frequency and haematuria, and toxicity is worse than the use of chemotherapy agents. Sepsis has been reported. Treatment with 300 mg isoniazid daily helps relieve the symptoms of chemotherapy toxicity. After BCG treatment for carcinoma in situ, 70% of patients may get a recurrence of their tumour after 10 years. Failed intravesical therapy may warrant a different intravesical agent as second line; however, this may be an indication for cystectomy.

In muscle invasive bladder cancer (T2–T4), radical cystectomy is the treatment of choice although radiotherapy is offered in selected cases, preserving the bladder. Neoadjuvant therapy is offered. The advantages of neoadjuvant therapy are that micrometastases may be treated and that there may be downstaging of the tumour before surgery (International Collaboration of Trialists 2000). A meta-analysis has shown some survival advantage using platinum-based chemotherapy (Advanced Bladder Cancer (ABC) Meta-analysis Collaboration 2003).

Adjuvant therapy has been used after surgery to help eliminate micrometastatic disease, although there is only a small amount of trial data available. Cyclophosphamide, cisplatin and doxorubicin combinations have been used. Typical regimens that have been used in the neoadjuvant setting include:

- CMV: cisplatin, methotrexate and vinblastine
- MVAC: methotrexate, vinblastine, doxorubicin and cisplatin
- GC: gemcitabine and cisplatin.

Chemotherapy is the mainstay of treatment in metastatic disease. Single-agent cisplatin therapy has given response rates of up to 65% but the prognosis remains poor, with the median survival being 3–6 months. The gold standard chemotherapy regimen is MVAC, with a near 40% complete response rate at the expense of toxicity and low long-term survival. Toxicity includes myelosuppression with sepsis. High-dose MVAC with G-CSF has shown better response rates with less toxicity. Similarly, new therapy agents have given high response rates and combination agents

Bladder cancer: case I

A 54-year-old man was referred to an urologist following two episodes of painless haematuria. An intravenous urogram (IVU) showed a large papillary tumour on the left side of the bladder. Following a transurethral resection of the bladder tumour, the histology was returned as a G3–T2 carcinoma. Histology confirmed this as a poorly differentiated transitional cell carcinoma with superficial muscle invasion. He was referred to a medical oncologist who advised three courses of neodjuvant MVAC chemotherapy followed by radiotherapy. Check cystoscopy after treatment completion indicated that the tumour was cleared and he remains well.

Comment

MVAC (the combination of methotrexate, vinblastine, doxorubicin and cisplatin) is used in the neoadjuvant and adjuvant setting in muscle invasive bladder cancer as well as in the palliative treatment of metastatic bladder cancer. This patient could have had cystectomy after neoadjuvant therapy as an option. Herr et al (1998) demonstrated that the majority of patients with invasive bladder tumours who achieve T0 status after neoadjuvant MVAC chemotherapy can preserve their bladders. This may be as long as 10 years after transurethral resection of the bladder tumour. However, there is a risk of new invasive tumours. Cystectomy is used to treat relapsed patients although the previous use of radiotherapy can make surgery technically difficult. The toxicities of treatment include significant myelosuppression, emesis and alopecia. There is a risk of cardiomyopathy, peripheral neuropathy, renal and otoxicity.

such as gemcitabine and cisplatin have progressed through Phase III trials showing similar response rates and survival to MVAC (Hussain & James 2003).

BREAST CANCER

In recent years, chemotherapy for the treatment of breast cancer has advanced through new drug development and clinical trial work. Tamoxifen has been shown to reduce the incidence of invasive and non-invasive breast cancer in high-risk women. Aromatase inhibitors are now available as the choice of treatment for secondary hormonal therapy in metastatic breast cancer. The use of chemotherapy such as doxorubicin and taxane in the adjuvant setting has been developed. New biological treatment using trastuzumab (Herceptin®) in patients who overexpress the HER2/neu oncogene opens up the opportunity to develop new drugs based on molecular targets. The use of biphosphonates for the treatment of metastatic bone disease is important in palliation of symptoms and confirmation that high-dose chemotherapy with peripheral stem-cell support has no advantage over standard therapy for metastatic breast cancer illustrates the importance of gathering the evidence from sound clinical trial work.

BREAST CANCER BIOLOGY

The natural history of breast cancer is directly related to the number of axillary nodes involved, this is the most important prognostic variable; 35–50% of patients are axillary node positive at the time of diagnosis, confirming the systemic nature of breast cancer.

Micrometastatic disease may be present in at least 50% of breast cancer patients at the time of diagnosis. Women with breast cancer lumps < 4 cm treated with lumpectomy, axillary dissection and primary breast irradiation have disease-free and overall survivals similar to modified radical mastectomy. This is clearly important in reducing morbidity, including psychological issues from having a radical mastectomy.

HORMONE RECEPTORS AND GROWTH FACTORS

The content of oestrogen and progesterone receptors within a breast cancer is important prognostically and is an indicator of response to endocrine therapy. Receptors correlate with various parameters related to cellular activity, such as turnover and histological differentiation. The fact that receptor-positive patients have longer disease-free intervals indicates the importance of assaying hormone receptors in breast tissue.

Growth factors such as epidermal growth factor, insulin-like growth factor and somatostatin have been identified within breast cancers. Oestrogen-negative tumours tend to have a higher level of epidermal growth factor receptor than oestrogen-positive tumours. Tumours with higher levels of epidermal growth factor tend to have poorer prognoses.

MOLECULAR TARGETS AND ONCOGENES

Epidermal growth factor is the gene product of the HER2/neu (erb B2) oncogene. Amplification of this oncogene correlates with prognosis in stage I and II breast cancers. Higher levels of HER2/neu have been shown to have shorter disease-free intervals and overall survival (Press 1997). Overexpression of HER2/neu predicts resistance to endocrine therapy and sensitivity to chemotherapy.

p53, a tumour suppressor gene, is linked to apoptosis. Loss of p53 may decrease the apoptotic potential of tumour cells and lose tumour suppression, leading to cellular proliferation of the cancer.

The c-myc oncogene is critical to the growth of human breast cancer cell lines and is directly regulated by ostrogens in hormone-dependent breast cancer cells. C-myc amplification occurs in 2–30% of patients with breast cancer and associated with poor prognosis. Women who carry mutations in either the BRCA1 or BRCA2 gene are at very high risk of developing both breast and ovarian cancers. No prospective data are yet available to indicate whether preventive hormonal therapy in these groups of women is beneficial.

ACTION OF HORMONES ON BREAST TISSUE

- Oestrogen: this is the main stimulus for growth of hormone-dependent breast cancer. Oestrogen is synthesised mainly in the ovary but also by the adrenal glands, adipose tissue and the breast tissue itself.
- Prolactin: acts with growth hormone to promote breast ductal development.
- Progesterone: acts with oestrogen and prolactin to promote lobuloalveolar development.

Historical ablative therapy such as adrenalectomy and hypophysectomy has been superseded by endocrine therapy.

Hormonal agents

Tamoxifen The use of adjuvant treatment with tamoxifen is dependent on the presence of oestrogen receptor in tumour cells and is a predictive factor for how patients might respond to tamoxifen. However, even in the presence of oestrogen-receptor-positive tumours, some patients with tumours do not respond or develop resistance to tamoxifen treatment. This reflects the heterozygous nature of the cancer biology of breast cancer. Fisher et al (1998) and the Early Breast Cancer Trialists' Collaborative Group (2001) confirmed the role of tamoxifen in the adjuvant setting in early breast cancer with a lowered incidence of contralateral breast cancer. Surgical excision with or without radiotherapy plus adjuvant tamoxifen will result in long-term disease-free survival for 80% of patients in early disease. Tamoxifen is the treatment of choice for postmenopausal women with hormonally responsive metastatic breast cancer. It is also considered primary treatment of choice in premenopausal women (Ingle et al 1986). It leads to a lower risk of recurrence in women with a history of lobular carcinoma in situ or atypical hyperplasia, as well as in women aged 35–59 years with a high predicted risk for breast cancer (Fisher et al 1998).

The biological effect is usually achieved with a dose of 20 mg once daily, although higher doses have been prescribed. The receptor status of the breast tumour predicts response rates. Thus patients with both oestrogen- and progesterone-positive receptor tumours can have response rates close to 80%, whereas patients with negative oestrogen and progesterone receptors may respond in less than 10% of cases.

Generally, surgery should be performed despite the age of patient. In elderly patients who are not good surgery cases, tamoxifen as primary treatment has led to a 27% complete response rate and a 60% total objective response rate. Overall survival is the same as in elderly woman treated with mastectomy, although the local recurrence rate in tamoxifen-treated patients is higher (Gaskell et al 1992).

Tamoxifen has a cytostatic action and works as a non-steroidal antioestrogen acting as an oestrogen agonist. It can bind reversibly with the oestrogen receptor and forms an inert complex that blocks oestrogen-mediated protein synthesis. It also has an effect on growth factors, blocking the production of the inhibitory growth factor TGF-β and the growth factors IGF-I and TGF-α.

Tamoxifen can prevent osteoporosis in postmenopausal women but may lead to bone loss in premenopausal women. Its side effects include hot flushes. Venlafaxine has been used to reduce this side effect (Loprinzi et al 2000). The use of hormone replacement therapy is generally not advocated in this setting. Through the HABITS trials, Holmberg et al (2004) demonstrated that new event breast cancers can occur if hormone replacement therapy is given after breast cancer diagnosis.

There is also an increased risk of thromboembolic disease by reducing levels of antithrombin III (Rutqvist & Mattsson 1993). The use of other selective oestrogen receptor modulators (SERMs) such as raloxifene and toremifene, also promotes deep vein thrombosis and none relieves the symptoms of the menopause. The increased risk of venous thromboembolism associated with tamoxifen is similar to that found for hormone replacement therapy. The absolute risk of deep venous thrombosis and pulmonary embolism is low in women under the age of 50.

> **Breast cancer: case 1**
>
> A 50-year-old woman presented to her GP with a breast lump above the left breast nipple and a 2-week history of bleeding from the nipple. She underwent surgical excision of the lump, which showed carcinoma; none of the axillary lymph nodes showed tumour involvement. The tumour was oestrogen-receptor-positive. In view of the presenting local tumour, she was offered postoperative radiotherapy followed by tamoxifen 20 mg for the next 5 years.

There is an increased risk of endometrial cancer, which tends to be low grade and surgically curable. The rates of endometrial cancer are higher in women aged 50 years or more and tend to be stage I localised disease. These women are also at risk of stroke, pulmonary embolism and deep vein thrombosis. Tamoxifen flare has been reported with bone and soft tissue pain in 10% of cases. This usually develops in the first few weeks of therapy. Generally, it reflects a response to treatment. The dose should be continued and the pain treated with analgesia or other symptomatic treatment. Hypercalcaemia has also been reported.

Most tumours tend to become refractory to the antiproliferative effects of tamoxifen between 2 and 5 years and 5 years of use is considered to be optimal. The role of new oestrogen receptor antagonists, such as fulvestrant, has been encouraging (Howell et al 2004), as have the aromatase inhibitors (Winer et al 2005).

Progestins The progestational agents such as megestrol acetate and medroxyprogesterone acetate have activity equivalent to that of tamoxifen in advanced hormonally responsive breast cancer in postmenopausal women. However, they are usually used as second or third line because their duration of response is slightly less than tamoxifen. Response rates after treatment failures with tamoxifen range from 14 to 22%, whereas only 14–22% of patients who are initially treated with these agents and then with tamoxifen respond. They act to inhibit oestrogen-induced protein synthesis. Weight gain is a problem with these agents and their appetite-stimulating effect is used to treat cancer anorexia and cachexia. Higher doses have been associated with arterial and pulmonary emboli.

Luteinising hormone-releasing hormone agonists LHRH analogues act on the pituitary, the gonads and the target sex organs. Examples are goserelin, buserelin and leuprorelin. Goserelin (Zoladex®) has an objective response rate of 45%, particularly in patients with loco-regional metastases. Side effects include amenorrhea, vaginal spotting, headache and sleep disturbance. In metastatic breast cancer in premenopausal women, goserelin has a response rate similar to ovariectomy. In postmenopausal women with oestrogen-receptor-positive tumours, the response rates have been at around 10%.

AROMATASE INHIBITORS

The enzyme aromatase converts androstenedione to oestrone, which is converted to oestradiol. Aromatase is present in adipose tissue, liver, muscle and breast tissue. The new aromatase inhibitors replace aminogluthemide, which blocked adrenal steroidogenesis but which had side effects. The types of aromatase inhibitor now available are the non-steroidal triazole inhibitors such as anastrazole, letrozole, vorozole and fadrozole and the steroidal aromatase inhibitors such as formestane and exemestane. The steroidal aromatase inhibitors bind irreversibly to aromatase, whereas the triazoles are reversible inhibitors. Because of their efficacy and lack of toxicity, these new aromatase inhibitors have emerged as the clear choice for secondary hormonal therapy after tamoxifen.

Baum et al (2003) reported the results of the Arimedex, Tamoxifen Alone or in Combination (ATAC) Trial, which demonstrated that, in adjuvant endocrine therapy for postmenopausal patients with early-stage breast cancer, anastrozole was superior to tamoxifen in terms of disease-free survival, time to recurrence and incidence of contralateral breast cancer.

The double-blind, randomised controlled trial by Coombes et al (2004) in postmenopausal women affected by breast cancer who are usually prescribed tamoxifen showed that after 2–3 years of use with tamoxifen and then switching to exemestane, women had fewer recurrences than women who stayed on 5 years of tamoxifen alone; they also had improved disease-free survival.

Goss et al (2003) showed that, compared with placebo, letrozole therapy after the completion of standard 5 years of tamoxifen treatment significantly improves disease-free survival in postmenopausal women with breast cancer. This trial was terminated after 2 years in view of the positive results. Anastrazole (Bonneterre et al 2000) and letrozole (Mouridsen et al 2001) are at least equivalent to tamoxifen in oestrogen-receptor-positive metastatic breast cancer and the incidence of thromboembolic events and vaginal bleeding with the new aromatase inhibitors is less than tamoxifen.

SYSTEMIC CHEMOTHERAPY IN THE ADJUVANT SETTING

In 1992, the Early Breast Cancer Trialists' Collaborative Group performed a systematic review of the randomised trials of treatment of early breast cancer by hormonal, cytotoxic or immune therapy. This involved analysing data on 75 000 women receiving treatment in the form of systemic adjuvant therapy in early breast cancer. It confirmed that the use of adjuvant chemotherapy with more than one agent gave a significant increase in absolute survival and recurrence-free survival, particularly in node-positive patients. Six months of

Breast cancer: case 2

A 35-year-old woman presented to her GP with a mobile lump situated in the left upper outer quadrant of the left breast. She was referred to the breast clinic and needle aspiration and cytology revealed cells consistent with a medullary carcinoma. This was confirmed as a solid lesion on mammogram. She underwent lumpectomy and lymph node dissection. The cancer was removed with good tumour margins. The lymph nodes were all clear and her staging was defined as T2 G1 N0 M0. Her oestrogen status was weakly positive and the progesterone receptor status was negative. She had no adjuvant radiotherapy or chemotherapy because it was felt she had an excellent prognosis.

Ten years later she presented with breast pain in the right breast. Mammogram showed microcalcification in the upper part of the breast and histology confirmed a high-grade ductal carcinoma in situ. She underwent mastectomy and six courses of adjuvant CMF chemotherapy. She tolerated her chemotherapy well apart from cutaneous and mucosal toxicity and pyridoxine was added to counteract the cutaneous toxicity. Her tumour was oestrogen-receptor-negative, progesterone-receptor-positive and HER2-negative. Her chemotherapy had led to a premature menopause and thus it was argued that she should go onto tamoxifen. She remains in remission.

Comment

This patient has a T2 tumour (which is tumour > 2 cm and < 5 cm) and was well differentiated (G1). This patient's treatment CMF regimen reflects the work of the Early Breast Cancer Trialists' Collaborative Group (2002), which has analysed the use of polychemotherapy and determined the advantage of using regimens such as CMF in terms of improved survival rates of over 40% at 15 years and over 35% relapse-free survival. The toxicities of treatment include myelosuppression, emesis, pronounced or total head hair loss, gastrointestinal side effects such as mucositis, infertility and the risk of secondary malignancy. The fact that this woman is young going onto tamoxifen may mean loss of bone density over time and this would need to be monitored.

treatment with multiple chemotherapy agents was no worse than 1 year of treatment in terms of survival, and the use of multiple agents was better than single-agent chemotherapy. Death rates were also reduced in premenopausal women.

In an update in 2002, the same group looked at women enrolled in randomised controlled trials who had received multiple chemotherapy agents, including the anthracyclines as adjuvant treatment, for early breast cancer. It concluded that using multiple chemotherapy agents produced an absolute improvement in mortality of between 7 and 11% in 10-year survival for women aged less than 50 years of age at presentation with early breast cancer, and of about 2–3% for those aged 50–69 years.

Common chemotherapy regimens include FEC (5-FU, epirubicin and cyclophosphamide) and CMF (cyclophosphamide, methotrexate, 5-FU). The use of postoperative chemotherapy and hormonal therapy has also conferred a beneficial effect. Results from the National Surgical Adjuvant Breast and Bowel Project B-16 (Fisher 1990) showed that in the adjuvant setting the addition of chemotherapy to long-term tamoxifen in postmenopausal women improved the overall survival and disease-free survival; tamoxifen commenced at the completion of chemotherapy.

CHEMOTHERAPY FOR METASTATIC BREAST CANCER

Systemic chemotherapy is the main treatment considered for patients with metastatic breast cancer. Combination cytotoxic regimens have been shown to lead to higher response rates and longer duration of response and survival compared to single agent treatment.

A European panel of cancer experts (Crown et al 2002) has looked at the factors that indicate when chemotherapy regimens should be considered for women who have metastatic disease. Some of the important variables were considered to be:

- the time to relapse after adjuvant therapy received
- the extent of metastatic disease
- age
- the HER2 status, which is a marker of prognosis.

The aim of treatment in metastatic disease is not curative intent but to optimise palliation of symptoms and maximise overall survival.

Anthracycline-based chemotherapy has shown higher overall response rates than non-anthracycline-containing regimens. This is associated with better progression and overall survival outcomes. Systematic reviews of randomised controlled trials have established anthracyclines as first-line chemotherapy for metastatic disease. However, an anthracycline-based regimen is limited because of the risk of cumulative cardiotoxicity. New non-anthracycline regimens are therefore needed for metastatic disease. Epirubicin-based chemotherapy is as effective as doxorubicin-based chemotherapy in terms of efficacy. Typical regimens include:

- AC: doxorubicin with cyclophosphamide
- EC: epirubicin with cyclophosphamide
- FAC: fluorouracil with doxorubicin and cyclophosphamide
- FEC: fluorouracil with epirubicin and cyclophosphamide.

Non-anthracycline regimens in the form of CMF (cyclophosphamide, methotrexate and fluorouracil) are used as first-line therapy. In patients who have had anthracycline-based adjuvant therapy, retreatment with an anthracycline-based regimen is possible on relapse providing the dose received is not more than 450–550 mg/m^2 of doxorubicin or 700–900 mg/m^2 of epirubicin and that there has been an extended disease-free period (i.e. > 12 months). Anthracyclines may be limited over time by inherent or drug-induced resistance and toxicity. Approaches to overcome this and improve the therapeutic index include anthracycline analogues and incorporation into drug delivery vehicles such as liposomes.

Usual second-line chemotherapy is paclitaxel or docetaxel (Taxotere®). The latter is a semi-synthetic taxane. It has activity in advanced breast cancer. Dose-limiting toxicity includes grade 3 or 4 neutropenia. Response rates vary depending on whether patients have had minimal re-pretreatment (up to 65%) or have been pretreated, with response rates as low as 19%. They have been given in combination with anthracyclines with some good response rates.

What happens when patients relapse after first- and second-line chemotherapy? The aim of treatment now would be to stabilise disease without compromising quality of life and to offer treatment that gives clinical benefit. An option for third-line therapy is gemcitabine, either as

---

Breast cancer: case 3

An 80-year-old woman presented with a clinical malignant tumour of her left breast, which was confirmed on biopsy. This did not respond to primary tamoxifen and so she underwent wide local excision followed by adjuvant radiotherapy. Six years later she presented with lymphoedema. A CT scan indicated a 3-cm left axillary node and pulmonary metastases. The tumour was oestrogen-receptor-negative. She underwent radiotherapy to the left axilla but presented 6 months later with chest wall skin nodules with ulceration. Hormone treatment was not indicated in view of her negative status. Her performance status was good and it was felt that palliative chemotherapy in the form of MM might help to alleviate her symptoms. She tolerated two courses well but died suddenly of a myocardial infarction.

Comment

In this case, the use of chemotherapy is purely palliative. The combination of mitoxantrone and methotrexate is useful in the elderly or frail patient because of its reduced toxicity profile, in particular reduced cardiac toxicity. Other combinations of treatment that have been used in the palliation of symptoms include AC (doxorubicin and cyclophosphamide) and FEC (5-fluorouracil, epirubicin and cyclophosphamide). However, these combinations cause severe alopecia and moderate myelosuppression, and are not recommended in the palliative setting if patients have had prior anthracyclines in view of the risk of cardiotoxicity. Single-agent capecitabine, docetaxel, paclitaxel and vinorelbine have all been used, with response rates as high as 50%.

Breast cancer: case 4

A 53-year-old woman presented with a 3-cm lump in the lower part of the right breast. She had an abnormal mammogram. Cytology of the lump revealed this to be malignant. A wide local excision with axillary dissection was performed. The histology was a grade 2 invasive ductal carcinoma with 50% of the lymph nodes involved. Her tumour status was oestrogen-negative. Some of the resection margins involved carcinoma. Mastectomy was offered, which the patient declined. The best option was felt to be adjuvant methotrexate and mitozantrone together with concomitant radiotherapy to reduce the risk of local relapse. The possible side effects were nausea and vomiting, malaise and myelosuppression, stomatitis and mild alopecia. She suffered nausea and vomiting with the second course of MM chemotherapy and this was controlled with nozinan and dexamethasone. She also suffered stomatitis, constipation and lethargy. Prior to her fifth course of MM chemotherapy she suffered neutropenia, necessitating a dose reduction. She also completed a radical course of radiotherapy to the left breast, which was tolerated well apart from mild erythema to the right breast.

Three months after completing chemotherapy she re-presented with a dry cough and dyspnoea on exertion. Chest X-ray was normal and oxygen saturations were 98% on air. The possibilities considered were thromboembolic disease, radiation pneumonitis, obstructive pulmonary disease and lymphangitis. She improved following a trial of steroids, which helped her symptoms. Subsequent V/Q scan and peak flows were normal. A CT scan showed postradiation changes in the right upper lobe. Her symptoms resolved with a reducing course of steroids.

She remained well thereafter and was in remission for a year until she re-presented with an axillary node, which on fine needle aspiration (FNA) was confirmed as a recurrence. It was recommended she have adjuvant AC chemotherapy after mastectomy and reconstruction. Her tumour status was oestrogen-receptor-negative. Her nausea and vomiting side effects on treatment were covered with granisetron and domperidone. After her first course of chemotherapy she developed neutropenia and had a dose reduction on subsequent courses. Other side effects suffered included constipation, mucositis and nausea. She managed to complete six courses of chemotherapy but required transfusion for anaemia. Two months later she developed recurrent metastatic disease with the development of a large right pleural effusion. This needed thoracic pleurodesis followed by six courses of capecitabine. However, 2 months later she presented as an emergency to her GP: she was breathless and was found to be in heart failure. Subsequent echocardiogram indicated a dilated poorly contracting left ventricle with an ejection fraction of 40%. This was felt to be due to cardiotoxicity secondary to anthracycline therapy. Her performance status gradually declined and it was felt that no further active therapy could be offered. She died peacefully at home with the support of her GP and the palliative care team.

continued on page 88

> **Breast cancer: case 4** *continued*
> **Comments**
> This case highlights the potential sequelae of cancer and the distressing complications of treatment that patients might experience. This woman experienced complications related to both radiotherapy and chemotherapy. The importance from the primary care perspective is to be supportive and help in the palliation of distressing symptoms, as well as watching for potential complications of treatment. The use of the 5-HT$_3$-receptor antagonist such as granisetron as antiemetic therapy has revolutionised the administration of highly emetogenic chemotherapy agents. Drugs that are moderately to severely emetogenic include the platinum agents (e.g. cisplatin and carboplatin), streptomycin, cyclophosphamide and doxorubicin.

monotherapy or in combination with vinorelbine or cisplatin. However, this combination produces myelosuppression. Other drugs include combinations of newer drugs with older drugs to enhance activity with more favourable toxicity, which includes combining infusional 5-FU and capecitabine. Response rates with third-line therapy tend to be low. Single-agent carboplatin is active in patients with previously untreated metastatic breast cancer, producing response rates of 20–35%.

NICE GUIDELINES AND BREAST CANCER

Use of taxanes
NICE has recommended that paclitaxel is to be used in the treatment of metastatic breast cancer if standard anthracycline-containing therapy has failed or is not indicated. Docetaxel (Taxotere®) is used in patients with locally advanced or metastatic breast cancer in whom previous regimens of chemotherapy have failed. For both drugs there have been randomised controlled trials demonstrating improved response and progression-free survival. Trials have also shown that toxicities do not lead to an adverse quality of life compared to standard therapy. The use of taxanes in the adjuvant setting is restricted to clinical trials.

Breast cancer and the use of tastuzumab
Breast tumours may contain an amplification of the human epidermal growth factor receptor (HER2), which causes overexpression of the HER2 protein and is associated with a worse prognosis. Immunohistochemistry is used to measure expression of the HER2 protein and women with metastatic breast cancer (stage IV) who overexpress HER2 have a poorer survival rate. Tastuzumab is a recombinant humanised monoclonal antibody that targets the HER protein. It is given intravenously and has cardiotoxicity as one of its main side effects. Anaphylaxis also been reported.

In oestrogen-receptor-positive patients hormonal therapy is indicated as first-line treatment for advanced (stage III) or metastatic disease (stage IV).

In oestrogen-receptor-negative patients, an anthracycline-containing regimen of a combination of CMF (cyclophosphamide, methotrexate and fluorouracil) is the usual first-line treatment. If first-line chemotherapy fails, NICE states that docetaxel or paclitaxel should be used.

NICE advises that trastuzumab can be used as monotherapy if tumours express HER2 and if the patient has received two chemotherapy regimens for metastatic breast cancer. Appropriate chemotherapy includes an anthracycline and a taxane, or hormonal therapy in suitable patients. The current recommendation is that trastuzumab is used in combination with paclitaxel in women with tumour expression of HER2 if they have not received chemotherapy for metastatic breast cancer and when anthracycline treatment is not appropriate. Randomised controlled trials have shown the combination results in longer times to disease progression, duration of response and longer median survival; quality of life was also better.

Capecitabine treatment of locally advanced or metastatic breast cancer

The NICE guidelines stipulate that, in locally advanced or metastatic disease, capecitabine in combination with docetaxel is used in patients in whom anthracycline-containing regimens have failed. Monotherapy use of capecitabine is recommended in patients with locally advanced or metastatic breast cancer if they have not already received it in combination therapy and where either an anthracycline- or taxane-containing regimen has failed or further anthracycline therapy is contraindicated. Tumour response rates from Phase II trials ranged from 15 to 28%.

HIGH-DOSE CHEMOTHERAPY FOR BREAST CANCER

Early non-randomised trials were initially encouraging about the use of high-dose chemotherapy, particularly for patients highly emetogenic with node-positive primary breast cancer (Giordano et al 2002). Patients' bone marrows were supported by colony stimulating factors. However, patients going through this treatment had up to a 20% chance of dying.

The rationale for high-dose chemotherapy with autologous bone marrow or stem-cell transplant was that this treatment may improve survival rates by permitting higher doses of adjuvant chemotherapy to be given. A meta-analysis by Farquhar et al (2003a) compared the effectiveness of high-dose chemotherapy and autograft versus conventional chemotherapy for women with early, poor-prognosis breast cancer. The results of this Cochrane Review indicated no statistically significant difference in overall survival between women who received high-dose chemotherapy with autograft and women who received conventional chemotherapy, either at 3 or 5 years. The conclusion was that there was insufficient evidence to support the routine use of high-dose chemotherapy with autograft for women with early, poor-prognosis breast cancer.

The same principle was applied in women with metastatic breast cancer. A Cochrane Review by Farquhar et al (2003b) compared the effectiveness of high-dose chemotherapy and autologous bone marrow or stem-cell transplantation with conventional chemotherapy for women with metastatic breast cancer. There was evidence that high-dose chemotherapy and autograft improved progression-free survival at 1 and 2 years' follow-up compared to conventional chemotherapy, although there was no evidence of benefit in overall survival.

BREAST CANCER IN MEN

This occurs infrequently and accounts for < 1% of all patients diagnosed with breast cancer. In men under the age of 40 the incidence of breast cancer does seem to be rising;however, the incidence does increase with age. The typical profile of a man with breast cancer is as follows (Perkins & Middleton 2003):

- median age 68 years
- more common to have ductal invasive cancers (80% of all tumours)
- 80% of breast cancers are oestrogen-receptor-positive
- can have high levels of oestrogen or oestrogen–androgen imbalances
- androgen and progesterone steroid receptor expression abnormalities such as in Kleinefelter's syndrome
- a family history of breast cancer in female relatives
- a painless subareolar mass.

Mutations in BRCA1 do not increase the risk of breast cancer in men, however BRCA2 mutations do appear to be a risk factor in men and the frequency of BRCA2 mutations are higher in families with a male affected by breast cancer.

The most important negative prognostic factors are lymph node involvement, larger tumour size and oestrogen-negative hormonal status of the tumour.

There is some evidence that men treated with adjuvant doxorubicin-based chemotherapy for stage II or III disease have survival rates exceeding 85%.

Patients with local disease are treated by radical mastectomy. Adjuvant hormonal therapy does lead to increased survival with drugs such as tamoxifen. Adjuvant chemotherapy has been given in limited studies indicating improved outcomes.

In metastatic disease, hormonal therapy remains the first choice treatment but there are recommendations that men with breast cancer should receive chemotherapy if they have positive nodes, tumours larger than 1 cm and hormone-receptor-negative metastasis together with hormonal therapy for 5 years. Response rates vary but can be around 40%.

CARCINOMA OF UNKNOWN PRIMARY TUMOURS

These account for 5% of all tumours. Extensive diagnostic investigation is uncomfortable for the patient and causes time and delay in treatment. With early start of chemotherapy, median survival has improved from 3–6 months to 1 year. Newer imaging techniques, e.g. breast MRI, PET and other nuclear medicine imaging techniques, give clues to the origin of the tumour. Usually the symptoms of disease depend where the tumour has metastasised. Histological assessment will guide treatment, with 60% of tumours being well differentiated or moderately differentiated adenocarcinoma and 30% being poorly differentiated carcinomas. Treatment is guided by histological assessment, clinical examination, biochemical markers (such as tumour markers) and site of involvement. A best guess is then made. For example, a young man with retroperitoneal disease and elevated serum α-fetoprotein (AFP) should be treated with extragonadal germ-cell tumour regimens.

A significant proportion of patients with adenocarcinoma will have treatment with 5-FU regimens for presumed gastrointestinal tract cancers; survival rates are poor in this group. In the presence of such uncertainty, these patients need psychological support.

CERVICAL CANCER

In the UK there are just over 1000 deaths a year from cervical cancer in the UK, with around 3000 cases per year. In the UK screening every 3 years is recommended for women between 25 and 59 years, and at 5-yearly intervals until 64 years. The staging of cervical cancer determines the type of treatment and early stage cancers are curable (Table 5.2).

Overall 5-year survival is around 60%, with stage I disease having 90% 5-year survival. The poor survival in stage IV disease of less than 10% illustrates how aggressive this tumour can be.

Stage IA is limited disease with very low incidence of metastasis. It is usually managed with cone biopsy or simple total hysterectomy.

Stage IB invasive cancer can be treated either by radical surgery (radical hysterectomy and pelvic lymph node dissection) or radical radiotherapy (external beam radiotherapy and bracytherapy).

The role of neoadjuvant chemotherapy, whereby chemotherapy is given before radiotherapy, has been used although randomised trials have shown inconsistent results (Thomas 1999). Meta-analysis has shown heterogeneity in the type of trials with variation in the dose intensity and length of

TABLE 5.2 Staging of cervical cancer (FIGO) (Reproduced with kind permission)

Stage	Description
Stage 0	Carcinoma in situ
Stage I	Invasive carcinoma confined to cervix
Stage IA	Invasive carcinoma identified microscopically
Further division into depth and width:	
Stage IB	Preclinical lesions greater than stage IA or clinical lesions confined to cervix
Further division by size:	
Stage II	Carcinoma extending beyond cervix but not to pelvic side wall; carcinoma involves vagina but not its lower third
Stage III	Carcinoma extending onto pelvic wall; on rectal examination no cancer free space between tumour and side wall. Tumour involves lower $\frac{1}{3}$ of vagina. Includes patients with hydronephrosis or non-functioning kidney
Stage IV	Carcinoma extends beyond true pelvis or clinically involves bladder mucosa or rectum. Stage IVB represents spread to distant organs

chemotherapy given. The rationale for use is that chemotherapy may reduce tumour bulk and thus improve control by radiotherapy or surgical resection. Micrometastatic disease may be better controlled, reducing recurrence in regional lymph nodes and further spread. Chemotherapy before radiotherapy may ensure that drug is delivered to the tumour through tumour vascularisation, which may be compromised by irradiation.

Randomised trials have reported on the role of chemotherapy and radiotherapy for locally advanced cervical cancer (stage IB–IVA). Trials have shown a highly significant reduction in the rate of cancer progression and a longer disease-free survival for patients receiving cisplatin-based chemotherapy (e.g. cisplatin alone, cisplatin and 5-FU or cisplatin, 5-FU and hydroxyurea) concurrent with radiotherapy (Thomas 1999, Williams 1999). This applies to all stages of locally advanced cervical cancer independent of the dose and schedule of radiotherapy regimen. There is an increase in bone marrow toxicity.

Only 20% of women who have stage IVB cancers survive longer than 2 years. These women could have chemotherapy with radiotherapy to control disease. For the majority of patients, treatment is palliative, although surgical resection of solitary lung metastases confers an increased survival rate. Complete response after chemotherapy is rare and response rates with single or combination chemotherapy ranges in Phase II trials from 10 to 40%. Cisplatin and paclitaxel combinations have given encouraging results, with over 30% partial responses. However, myelosuppression remains a toxic side effect and quality of life is important in this group of patients. The chances of a response diminished if recurrence is within an irradiated area.

SUMMARY

There is clear evidence from randomised controlled trials that concurrent chemoradiotherapy using cisplatin improves survival in women with high-risk cervical cancer. Toxicity may be increased as a result. In women with stage Ib to IVa disease with locally advanced disease, involved lymph nodes or parametrial invasion, survival rates at 3 years increased by close to 50% for those women treated with cisplatin and radiotherapy.

COLORECTAL CANCER

Colorectal cancer accounts for the second most common cause of death in the UK from cancer, causing around 16 000 deaths per year. The molecular biology of colorectal cancer has been well defined and it is clear that there is a natural transition from normal to an adenoma and then carcinoma. This involves a sequence of genetic mutations. Mutations in the tumour suppressor genes APC, the K-ras proto-oncogene and the DCC tumour suppressor gene have been implicated.

STAGING OF COLORECTAL CANCER

Dukes' staging is used as an indicator of prognosis in the management of these patients:

- Dukes' A tumours: do not reach the bowel wall and there is no lymphatic involvement; 5-year survival is over 90%.
- Dukes' B tumours: reach the mesorectal or pericolic fat and have a 5-year survival of over 60%.
- Dukes' C tumours: have regional involvement and 5-year survival is just over 20%.
- The TNM staging system for colorectal cancer stages the cancer based on the degree of spread of local tumour, the presence of involved regional lymph nodes and the presence of metastases.
- Stage I tumours: equate to Dukes' A staging if there is no spread beyond the muscularis propria.
- Stage II tumours: equate to Dukes' B if there is no regional involvement and no distant metastases but the tumour has invaded the peritoneum or there is direct invasion of organs.
- Stage III tumours: equate to Dukes' C if there is nodal involvement without distant metastases.
- Stage IV tumours: equate to metastatic Dukes' D disease.

Surgery is the treatment of choice for the curative treatment of colorectal cancer with chemotherapy and radiotherapy being used for adjuvant therapy and the treatment of metastatic disease.

THE ROLE OF 5-FLUOROURACIL

The mainstay of chemotherapy treatment has been the use of 5-FU both in the adjuvant setting and in metastatic disease. The method of delivery of the drug varies:

- i.v. bolus for 5 days every 4–5 weeks
- a weekly single i.v. bolus
- continuous intravenous infusion.

One of the actions of the 5-FU and folinic acid combination is the inhibition of DNA synthesis. Although the continuous infusion regimen has shown better response rates than the i.v. bolus regimen, no significant difference in terms of time to progression and survival is evident from meta-analysis. The continuous infusion regimen suffers from a greater degree of haematological toxicity and the hand–foot syndrome, characterised by erythema, is more evident. The type of regimens used are the:

- Mayo Clinic regimen: the bolus 5-FU and folinic acid regimen of 5-FU 425 mg/m^2/day i.v. days 1–5 and leucovorin 20 mg/m^2/day i.v. days 1–5, both repeated every 4–5 weeks for 6 months.
- De Gramont regimen: leucovorin 200 mg/m^2 as a 2-hour infusion days 1 and 2. 5-FU 400 mg/m^2 i.v. then 5-FU 600 mg/m^2 continuous infusion over 22 hours days 1 and 2. Repeated every 14 days.
- Lokich regimen: 5-FU 300 mg/m^2/day by continuous i.v. infusion until toxicity or disease progression.

ADJUVANT CHEMOTHERAPY

Adjuvant chemotherapy with 5-FU regimens improves disease-free survival and overall survival times in patients with surgically resected stage III and some stage II (B2, B3) colon cancers and in patients with advanced disease:

- A 6-month course of chemotherapy with 5-FU and folinic acid has been shown to prolong survival. The regimen (Mayo Clinic regimen) is based on a daily i.v. bolus of folinic acid followed by an i.v. bolus of 5-FU for 5 days; repeated every 25 days.
- There is some debate about the role of adjuvant therapy in Dukes' B cancers and, to date, a significant survival benefit after administering 5-FU chemotherapy has not been proven.

ADVANCED METASTATIC DISEASE

Combinations of 5-FU and leucovorin have given response rates of up to 40%. A meta-analysis of randomised trials has shown the advantage of this combination over 5-FU alone in terms of reducing tumour bulk in advanced colorectal cancer (Benson 2004), although there does not appear to be a higher survival benefit. The use of neoadjuvant therapy in the presence of liver

Colorectal cancer: case 1

A 60-year-old man presented with a 7-week history of a change in bowel habit with loose motions up to four times daily. He was referred to a gastroenterologist by his GP. A colonoscopy was performed, which showed a transverse colon tumour. He underwent a right hemicolectomy and subsequent histology confirmed a poorly differentiated mucinous Dukes' B adenocarcinoma with no nodal involvement. He was then referred to oncology. It was recommended that he have 6 months of adjuvant chemotherapy with 5-FU and leucovorin by the Mayo Clinic regimen starting within 12 weeks of resection. His postoperative levels of carcinoembryonic antigen (CEA; a tumour marker) were normal. After cycle I of chemotherapy he developed grade II stomatitis and neutropenia with a white cell count (WCC) of 3.1. Cycle III was administered with a 25% dose reduction. He tolerated the rest of his chemotherapy without problem and postoperative CT scan and CEA showed he had no active disease. He underwent a surveillance colonoscopy 1 year after resection, which showed no active disease and he remains well under follow-up.

Comments

- The reason for recommending adjuvant chemotherapy in this man was that his histology of a poorly differentiating mucinous tumour is a poor prognostic factor.
- In the adjuvant setting there is a reduced recurrence rate and improved survival in patients treated with this combination of drugs. The same regimen is also used in the treatment of advanced colorectal cancer and in rectal cancer.
- The drop in white cell count illustrates how important it is to monitor for nadir counts. The cumulative effect of chemotherapy on bone marrow means that, without a dose reduction, this patient would have developed a serious neutropenia with potential for sepsis, which in the adjuvant setting could be disastrous. Most centres would dose reduce if WCC = 3.0×10^9/L and platelet count = 100×10^9/L or less.
- Another reason to delay treatment would be if this patient developed serious (grade 2 or higher) mucositis and diarrhoea. Some patients need i.v. hydration if the gastrointestinal symptoms are serious. The importance of oral hygiene should be imparted to the patient and mouthwashes, sucking ice-chips and, if necessary, antifungals help to reduce the effects of mucositis.
- Other side effects this patient might have experienced include vomiting, alopecia (usually grade 1), chest pain caused by 5-FU-induced coronary spasm, plantar–palmar syndrome and conjunctivitis. Plantar–palmar syndrome is associated with an erythematous rash, pain, swelling, tingling and desquamation of the skin distributed in those areas. It is an idiosyncratic reaction associated with 5-FU, capecitabine and continuous infusion doxorubicin. It is not associated with the type of disease or the amount of 5-FU given and a dose reduction usually resolves it. It needs good hand and foot care, analgesia and emollients: pyridoxine is also used to treat it.

continued on page 96

Colorectal cancer: case 1 *continued*
- CEA is a glycoprotein tumour marker that can be used to measure response to treatment if elevated before surgery or chemotherapy. It is associated with colorectal cancer but also is elevated in cancers of the stomach, pancreas and ovarian cancers. It can be elevated in non-cancerous conditions such as inflammatory bowel disease and pancreatitis.

Colorectal cancer: case 2

A 60-year-old man had an AP resection following the discovery of a carcinoma in the distal rectum. He had had 3 months of a change in bowel habit. The tumour was a Dukes' C adenocarcinoma of the distal rectum with only one out of 10 lymph nodes sampled being positive. He was advised to have adjuvant chemotherapy with 5-FU and folinic acid and completed six cycles. The main side effects he experienced were grade 2 stomatitis (treated with sucralfate) and grade 1 palmar–plantar erythema (treated with pyridoxine). Other side effects included alopecia. CT scan, tumour markers (CEA) and colonoscopy after completion of treatment showed no evidence of recurrent disease.

Comments

Oral complications are a common side effect associated with chemotherapy (Mead 2002). They can lead to dose reduction of effective chemotherapy. Patients are at risk of oral mucositis, infection, salivary gland dysfunction, trismus and taste alterations. The common chemotherapy drugs that cause these type of side effects are 5-FU, bleomycin, doxorubicin and methotrexate. Pain, weight loss with decreased intake and, in severe cases, an increased risk of sepsis are possible sequelae. Patients can suffer from nutritional deficiencies and abnormal dental development. Good oral hygiene, sucking ice chips, pilocarpine tablets and sucralfate are used to prevent mucositis. For established mucositis, antiseptic mouth washes and anti-inflammatory mouth washes have been prescribed, although some studies have suggested that these measures may worsen the pain associated with mucositis.

It may be that in the future new drugs such as capecitabine, oxaliplatin and irinotecan replace 5-FU as the gold standard in the adjuvant setting. The X-ACT Study Group provided some evidence that capecitabine has the potential to replace 5-FU/leucovorin as standard adjuvant treatment for patients with colon cancer. This trial compared adjuvant oral capecitabine with 5-FU and leucovorin (the Mayo Clinic regimen) in Dukes' C colon cancer. Patients who had resection of Dukes' C colon carcinoma were randomised to receive 6 months with either oral capecitabine 1250 mg/m^2 twice daily, days 1–14 every 21 days or an i.v. bolus of 5-FU 425 mg/m^2 with i.v. leucovorin 20 mg/m^2 on days 1–5, repeated every 28 days. It demonstrated that the 3-year relapse-free survival was better for capecitabine (65.5%) than for 5-FU (61.9%). The overall 3-year survival was 81.3% for capecitabine compared to 77.6% for 5-FU. The group also reported

Colorectal cancer: case 2 *continued*

safety data from a Phase III trial comparing the use of adjuvant oral capecitabine with the Mayo Clinic regimen in Dukes' C colon cancer (Scheithauer 2003). Patients receiving capecitabine experienced significantly fewer gastrointestinal side effects but more palmar–plantar syndromes.

The MOSAIC trial compared infusional 5-FU with leucovorin and oxaliplatin (FOLFOX-4) against 5-FU and leucovorin alone as adjuvant therapy in patients with stage II and III cancers. This trial showed that FOLFOX-4 had improved progression-free survival in node-positive patients over 5-FU/leucovorin alone. In stage II patients there was a risk reduction of 18% for patients who had received FOLFOX-4, with 3-year disease-free survivals of 86.6% versus 83.4% respectively, whereas for stage III disease there was a risk reduction of 24% with disease-free survivals of 71.8% versus 65.5% at 3 years.

metastases is being evaluated. Surgical resection of liver metastases is beneficial in only a small group of patients. The principle of using neoadjuvant chemotherapy is to reduce the size of liver metastases to enable surgical resection. Encouraging results are being seen with combinations of 5-FU and leucovorin with oxaliplatin followed by surgical resection of liver tumour.

NICE guidelines

Oxaliplatin This is a platinum-based compound that prevents DNA replication and leads to cell death. It can be used as first-line treatment in combination with 5-FU and folinic acid in patients with advanced colorectal cancer with liver metastases. Oxaliplatin can be used in patients with advanced colorectal cancer who have relapsed after 5-FU chemotherapy. Response rates have been as high as 50% and have been higher in untreated patients. It is given as an i.v. infusion. The main side effect of treatment is dose-limiting peripheral neuropathy. Randomised controlled trials have shown an increase in median progression-free survival by 2 months using oxaliplatin in combination with 5-FU and folinic acid, compared to 5-FU and folinic acid alone.

Irinotecan (CPT-11, Campto®) This is a topoisomerase I inhibitor. The drug is administered as a drug infusion. It is used in first-line chemotherapy in combination with 5-FU and folinic acid in advanced colon cancer. Phase II trials have shown an increase in progression-free survival by 2 months. It is used as monotherapy second-line chemotherapy in patients who have progressed following treatment with a 5-FU-containing regimen. Response rates can be around 15%, which is better than supportive care. Side effects of treatment include severe diarrhoea, myelosuppression, alopecia and acute cholinergic symptoms. In advanced disease, irinotecan can produce a better quality of life than best supportive care.

Capecitabine and tegafur Capecitabine is a prodrug that is taken orally. It is metabolised to fluorouracil and is given as monotherapy for metastatic colorectal cancer and breast cancer.

Tegafur is a fluropyrimidine taken orally. It is a prodrug of fluorouracil. It is taken in combination with uracil and calcium folinate; the uracil inhibits the degradation of fluorouracil. It is used in the management of metastatic colorectal cancer. Compared with 5-FU and folinic acid, the combination is not statistically different in terms of clinical effectiveness. Capecitabine has a better response rate but no significant differences in progression-free or overall survival times than standard 5-FU and folinic acid in Phase III randomised trials. Capecitabine had better-tolerated toxicity profiles with less gastrointestinal toxicity and was better tolerated overall in view of the fact it is taken orally. Phase II studies evaluating the combinations of capecitabine and oxaliplatin, and oxaliplatin and irinotecan in colorectal cancer have found good response rates.

Ralitrexed This drug is a thymidylate synthase inhibitor, an enzyme critical for DNA synthesis. It is used as palliative treatment for advanced colorectal cancer if 5-FU- and folinic-acid-based regimens are not recommended. It is given as an i.v. infusion. It should be used as part of a clinical trial only.

Colorectal cancer: case 3

An 80-year-old man presented to his GP with a history of rectal bleeding and abdominal discomfort on the right side of his abdomen. He was also found to be anaemic. Following referral to a colorectal surgeon, subsequent colonoscopy revealed a large polypoid cancer in the ascending colon and caecum. He underwent hemicolectomy. Histology and CT scan of the abdomen showed this tumour to be a Dukes' B adenocarcinoma staged as T4 N0. He was seen by a medical oncologist who felt that, in view of his age, the risks and toxicities of chemotherapy would outweigh any benefit to him.

Colorectal cancer: case 4

A 75-year-old man presented to his GP with rectal bleeding. On rectal digital examination a firm mass was palpable. He was referred to a colorectal surgeon. The tumour was biopsied and histology revealed this to be an adenocarcinoma. The tumour was 4 mm above the dentate line and it was felt that sphincter-sparing surgery would be difficult. The tumour was staged as T2 N0 stage I. He was referred to a cancer centre and his oncologist proceeded with a course of chemoradiotherapy prior to an AP resection. He was put onto a Phase II trial, which was evaluating the efficacy and toxicity of the combination of two drugs (capecitabine with a platinum agent) followed by radiotherapy. He suffered symptoms, including hand–foot syndrome, diarrhoea and bone marrow suppression through his course of chemotherapy. He managed to complete treatment with an excellent response and tolerated his AP resection.

continued on page 99

Colorectal cancer: case 4 *continued*
Comment

Clinical studies have shown the benefit of preoperative chemoradiotherapy with 5-FU-based regimens in rectal cancer (Madoff 2004). This has led to reductions in local recurrences and improved survival and led to sphincter preservation. 5-year survival rates of over 70% with relapse-free survival rates close to 80% have been reported with 5-FU and leucovorin treatment in patients with stage II and III cancers. The advantage of 5-FU chemoradiotherapy is that it results in improved organ preservation, including head and neck cancer, anal and rectal cancers, with improved sphincter preservation (Rich 2004). 5-FU has been the standard drug used in combination with radiation therapy but, more recently, new drugs such as capecitabine, oxaliplatin and irinotecan are being studied in combination with radiotherapy in the preoperative setting.

ENDOMETRIAL CANCER

Endometrial cancer accounts for over 5000 new cases a year in the UK, with 75% occurring in postmenopausal women. The endometrium is responsive to oestrogen and chronic unopposed oestrogenic stimulation can lead to endometrial cancers. Over 90% of endometrial cancers are adenocarcinomas and clear-cell cancers as described in the case study above tend to be rarer. This patient has local disease with an approximately 30% chance of recurrence. Tumour grade, G1–G3 with grade 3 being poorly differentiated tumour is important, with the higher grade having an increased risk of local recurrence. Most patients present with stage I disease and the overall 5-year survival rate is 75%. This patient had an intermediate risk of recurrence based on the fact that she had myometrial invasion and was graded as IB. The staging of endometrial cancer is as described by the FIGO (Fédération Internationale de Gynécologie et d'Obstétrique) staging system (Jones 2002) (Table 5.3).

Endometrial cancer: case 1

A 65-year-old woman had two episodes of postmenopausal bleeding. She underwent a hysteroscopy, which showed three endometrial polyps in the fundal area of the uterus, so she underwent endometrial polypectomy with a dilatation and curettage (D&C). Her histology came back as a poorly differentiated predominantly clear-cell endometrial carcinoma. An MRI scan showed that the disease was confined to the uterus. She underwent an extended hysterectomy and bilateral salpingo-oophorectomy as part of a randomised trial comparing to standard treatment.

continued on page 100

Endometrial cancer: case I *continued*

Her histology demonstrated a high-grade serous papillary/clear-cell tumour G3 with superficial myometrial invasion to a depth of 1 mm with lymphovascular invasion. There was no involvement of the cervix, fallopian tubes or ovaries.

She received adjuvant pelvic radiotherapy. She developed severe hot flushes and sweats, which necessitated the commencement of hormone replacement therapy (HRT). It was felt that she needed an opposed oestrogen preparation to help her menopausal symptoms and because of the theoretical risk of residual microscopics, endometrial cancer being stimulated by exogenous oestrogens. She was advised that she did not need vault smears because these are of little predictive value in the follow-up of patients with endometrial cancer. She remains in remission.

TABLE 5.3 Staging of endometrial cancer (FIGO)

Stage	Description
I A	Endometrial disease only
I B	Inner half of myometrium affected
I C	Outer half of myometrium affected
IIA	Extension to the endocervical glandular area
IIB	Invasion of the cervical stroma
IIIA	Invasion to one or more of the serosa, adnexa or peritoneum
IIIB	Invasion of the pelvic or para-aortic lymph nodes
IV	Involvement of one or more of bladder, bowel, inguinal nodes, abdominal or distant metastases

Surgery such as total abdominal hysterectomy and bilateral salpingo-oophorectomy and radiotherapy are the treatment modalities of choice. The rationale for this patient to have adjuvant treatment after surgery was the involvement of the myometrial and the purpose of this treatment is to prevent local recurrence. Chemotherapy and hormonal therapy have not been shown to improve survival in this group of patients.

A trial by the Clinical Outcomes Group (COG; Keys et al 2004) showed that patients receiving radiotherapy after total hysterectomy and bilateral salpingo-oophorectomy had a reduced relapse rate and a good 2-year progression-free survival compared with patients who receive no radiotherapy. Radiotherapy does make the use of vault smears as a means of monitoring for relapse difficult to interpret.

Chemotherapy has been used in advanced stage IV disease, with doxorubicin giving the best response rates (up to 50%) in combination with cisplatin. Other agents that have been tried include paclitaxel, although responses are low and a matter of few months.

Endometrial cancer: case 2

A 55-year-old postmenopausal woman was treated with neoadjuvant AC chemotherapy with a complete response for a left inflammatory breast cancer. This was followed by radiotherapy and then tamoxifen for 5 years. She presented to her GP with a history of vaginal bleeding and a transvaginal scan by a gynaecologist revealed a thickened endometrium of 14 mm. Hysteroscopy revealed an irregular polypoid mass within the endometrial cavity and biopsy confirmed this as a mixed Mullerian tumour of the endometrium. An MRI scan confirmed bilateral pelvic lymphodenopathy and enlargement of the endometrial cavity. She was staged as IIIc. She underwent total abdominal hysterectomy, bilateral salpingo-oophorectomy and pelvic lymphadenectomy. At surgery it was noted that she had para-aortic nodal disease, which was a contraindication for adjuvant radiotherapy. It was felt that she would benefit from carboplatin and paclitaxel chemotherapy. Anthracycline chemotherapy would be contraindicated in view of her previous treatment regimen. The potential side effects of this treatment were hypersensitivity reactions, myelosuppression, infection, alopecia and peripheral neuropathy. Ten minutes into the paclitaxel infusion she developed an allergic reaction and so was able to receive only single-agent carboplatin. However, after three courses of treatment she developed progressive retroperitoneal disease, her performance status fell to 2 and it was felt that she would be better treated through the palliative care team.

Comments

A recent population-based study looking at long-term survivors of breast cancer has shown that the use of tamoxifen is associated with an overall four-fold relative risk for mixed Mullerian tumour, although the absolute risk of death is small (Rochelle 2004). A meta-analysis (Braithwaite 2003) has shown that tamoxifen use is associated with significantly increased risks of endometrial cancer, with a significant relative risk of 2.70. The development of uterine pathology over time will be reported in the use of tamoxifen in the ATAC study. There is no consensus for a surveillance protocol for women on tamoxifen. Patients must be warned about vaginal bleeding or any other new gynaecological symptoms.

Endometrial tumours do carry oestrogen and progesterone receptors and in those patients with advanced disease, such as stage IV disease, progesterone therapy such as with the use of oral medroxyprogesterone has been used. Response rates are as low as 20%. In the small subgroup of patients who develop uterine sarcoma, the use of progesterones in the presence of metastatic disease has given good response rates.

GASTRIC CANCER

In the UK the incidence of gastric cancer is around 10 000 new cases per year. The highest incident rates are in Japan and China, although the incidence of gastric cancer and mortality rates are falling worldwide as a result of nutritional improvements in diet. In Japan, screening has improved survival with detection rates of 40%. In early gastric cancer, 5-year survival is higher than 90%. However, in the UK the most common presentation tends to be with locally advanced disease (Table 5.4) and median survival rates fall to 30% because of systemic metastases, which usually occur in people aged over 55 years.

The predominant histological type is adenocarcinoma. In early-stage disease and locally advanced disease, surgery either as a subtotal gastrectomy or total gastrectomy with distal oesophagectomy is considered and offers the only potential curative treatment.

Neoadjuvant chemotherapy to downstage the tumour has not been encouraging, even with combined modality treatment of chemotherapy

TABLE 5.4 TNM staging of gastric cancer

Grade	Description
Tumour (T)	
Tis	Carcinoma in situ
T1	Tumour invades lamina propria or submucosa
T2	Tumour invades muscularis propria or subserosa; extension into omenta or gastrohepatic ligaments
T3	Tumour penetrates serosa
T4	Tumour invades adjacent structures
Lymph node (N)	
N0	No regional lymph-node metastases
Nx	Less than 15 investigated lymph nodes (usually examine > 15)
N1	1–6 regional lymph-node metastases
N2	7–15 regional lymph-node metastases
N3	More than 15 regional lymph-node metastases
Metastases (M)	
M0	No distant metastases
M1	Distant metastases

and radiotherapy. Meta-analysis has shown no evidence that postoperative adjuvant chemotherapy makes any difference to survival (Hermans 1993).

Thus chemotherapy is used largely in the palliative care setting in advanced disease. 5-FU is the mainstay chemotherapy agent of choice although there are relatively low response rates and poor survival using 5-FU alone, which has led to combining 5-FU with other agents with little clinical benefit. Phase II trials have shown good response rates although the results in well-controlled randomised trials have not been encouraging. Combinations in advanced unresectable gastric cancer (Webb 1997) include:

- ECF: epirubicin, cisplatin and continuous infusion 5-FU
- FAMTX: 5-FU, doxorubicin and high-dose methotrexate (Table 5.5)
- ELF: etoposide, folinic acid (leucovorin) and 5-FU.

Response rates with the epirubicin, cisplatin and infusional 5-FU (ECF combinations) have been encouraging (up to 50%) with survival rates better than supportive care, i.e. up to 12 months with chemotherapy against 5 months with supportive care (Chau 2004). The 5-year survival for stage IV cancers is less than 5%.

Newer agents, such as irinotecan and oxaliplatin, have been through clinical trials in gastric cancer and offer some potential (Diaz-Rubio 2004). As a single agent, irinotecan (a potent topoisomerase I inhibitor) has shown response rates of 18–43%. In combination regimens with 5-FU and cisplatin, particularly in chemotherapy-naïve patients, irinotecan produced response rates up to 59%. Further trial results are awaited. Similarly, oxaliplatin, a new platinum analogue, has gone through Phase II studies having shown potential in gastric cancer therapy when combined with 5-FU and folinic acid.

The taxane docetaxel has also been shown to have activity in gastric cancer. As a single agent, docetaxel achieved response rates of 20–24%. Docetaxel combinations with other drugs have also demonstrated significant activity in gastric cancer, although toxicity, particularly neutropenia, remains dose limiting.

In summary, there is no standard chemotherapeutic regimen for gastric cancer. Current therapies offer some benefit in terms of palliation and survival but the benefit is small.

TABLE 5.5 Comparison of ECF and FAMTX regimens

	Overall response rate (%)	Median survival (months)	2-year survival (%)
ECF	46	8.	14
FAMTX	21	6.1	5

Gastric cancer: case 1

A 65-year-old woman presented with a history of around 14.5-kg weight loss associated with anorexia, early satiety and vomiting. She was referred for an upper GI endoscope and gastric biopsies confirmed gastric adenocarcinoma linitus plastica, with the laparoscope confirming omental adenocarcinoma. Her disease status did not make her amenable to surgical treatment and thus was referred for consideration of chemotherapy. ECF chemotherapy was recommended.

Comments

ECF treatment incorporates epirubicin, cisplatin and 5-FU. The toxicities of this regimen include severe emesis and hair loss, myelosuppression, gastrointestinal symptoms such as diarrhoea, neurotoxicity, renal toxicity, ototoxicity and cardiac toxicity. The last is associated with cumulative doses of epirubicin and monitoring of left ventricular ejection fraction is necessary. The median survival time is likely to be around 8 months in this case. This is better than supportive care alone. New drug combinations such as capecitabine and oxaliplatin are going through Phase II trials. The use of 5-FU with leucovorin is used in patients with poor performance status.

GESTATIONAL TROPHOBLASTIC DISEASE

Gestational trophoblastic disease (GTD) forms a spectrum of cancer diagnosis from the molar pregnancy to invasive mole and choriocarcinoma. Due to advances in the management of these malignancies, cure is highly likely and the role of chemotherapy is important.

The diagnosis is made if, after the removal of a hydatidiform mole, there is:

- rising human chorionic gonadotrophin (hCG) levels
- histology showing an invasive mole or choriocarcinoma.

The diagnosis is also made if, after pregnancy, there is a persistently elevated hCG level.

Classification of the extent of disease can be at three levels and is dependent on the use of biochemical markers, such as measurement of hCG, and scans, such as CT and MRI, to document extent of disease spread. The three levels of disease are:

- non-metastatic disease
- low-risk metastatic disease
- high-risk metastatic disease.

The staging system for GTD (Bloss & Thigpen 2001) takes this risk assessment into account as shown in Table 5.6.

TABLE 5.6 Staging for gestational trophoblastic disease (GTD)

Stage	Extent of disease	Risk assessment
0	Molar pregnancy	Non-metastatic disease
I	GTD confined to uterine corpus	Low risk unless have factors
II	GTD metastases to vagina and pelvis	High risk*
III	GTD metastases to lungs	High risk*
IV	Distant metastases	High risk*

* Factors determining a high risk include urinary hCG > 100 000 IU/24 hours, time before treatment > 4 months, term pregnancy, other sites of metastases, prior unsuccessful pregnancy.
Note: All patients should be registered at a trophoblastic centre.

In non-metastatic disease, hysterectomy and single-agent chemotherapy with methotrexate and folic acid is the standard treatment. Actinomycin-D is an alternative and results in 85–90% cure rates. In those who want to preserve fertility, hysterectomy should be reconsidered if hCG levels plateau or rise after two courses of treatment and the other single agent used.

In low-risk metastatic disease, a single-agent chemotherapy agent (as above) should be used, although 50% of patients may develop resistance and will need a change to the other single agent. Ten to fifteen per cent of patients may require combination chemotherapy, possibly with surgery. Monitoring for changes in hCG and new metastases are important.

In high-risk metastatic disease, only 20% of patients respond to single-agent therapy; combination therapies lead to cure rates of 80%, although these patients are at risk of brain and hepatic metastases. Secondary malignancies that occur after the treatment of these patients include myeloid leukaemia and have been associated with the use of etoposide. The type of chemotherapy commonly given in the UK is:

- EMACO: etoposide, actinomycin-D, methotrexate, vincristine and cyclophosphamide (Newlands et al 1999a).

Patients with relapsing or resistant disease can be treated either with surgery or surgery plus cisplatin in EP/EMA (etoposide, platinum-etoposide, methotrexate, actinomycin-D) leading to 80% complete remission rates (Newlands et al 1999b).

GLIOMAS

The classification of brain tumours is based on their tissue of origin; the World Health Organization classification system is the most widely used. The most common brain tumours are gliomas and meningiomas.

In adults, gliomas, which are tumours of neuroepithelial tissue, peak between the ages of 50 and 60 years. The incidence of gliomas is around 10 per 100 000 of the general population. There are three main types of glioma:

- astrocytomas (which account for 80% of gliomas)
- oligodendrogliomas
- mixed oligoastrocytomas.

Familial genetic disorders (e.g. neurofibromatosis type 1) are associated with gliomas. Gliomas tend to be infiltrating, which makes resection difficult and usually results in severe morbidity with neurological damage. The usual treatment is surgery to minimise tumour bulk followed by radiotherapy. The median survival time is around 9 months and only 5–10% survive to 2 years. Chemotherapy is used from the neoadjuvant setting through to palliative care (Rampling 2002).

The histological grade is important for determining prognosis with high-grade gliomas. The histological presence of a glioblastoma (a poorly differentiated astrocytic tumour) makes a tumour a high-grade stage IV glioma. Surgery and postoperative radiotherapy is the mainstay of treatment. It has been shown that maximal debulking produces longer survival rate than resections. There have been reported increases in survival following surgery compared with palliative care alone. Postoperative radiotherapy again leads to an increase in median survival. However, the outlook still is poor in these high-grade tumours, with a median survival of less than 1 year.

The use of adjuvant chemotherapy is debatable and there is evidence that perhaps chemotherapy should be used for tumour recurrence rather than as adjuvant therapy. A recent systematic review and meta-analysis to assess the value of systemic chemotherapy showed a small but significant improvement in survival in patients with high-grade gliomas (Glioma Meta-analysis Trialists' Group 2002). In this systematic review of patients with high-grade gliomas, patients were randomised to radiotherapy or radiotherapy with chemotherapy. There was an increase of 6% in the 1-year survival (from 40% to 46%) in the chemotherapy arm, with a 2-month increase in median survival.

Drugs that were found to be active in brain tumours include the nitrosoureas (e.g carmustine and lomustine), procarbazine, temozolamide, cisplatin and etoposide. In relapsed glioma the standard chemotherapy combination therapy used is PCV (procarbazine, CCNU and vincristine). Side effects include myelosuppression, emesis, pulmonary fibrosis, neuropathy and renal and hepatic toxicity. There is little difference compared to some single-agent chemotherapy regimens. Temozolamide has shown good activity in malignant glioma. In Phase II trials it showed single-agent activity of over 50% in terms of 1-year survival with a good quality of life. Side effects include myelosuppression and emesis. The use of combination chemotherapy in these tumours does not seem to confer any great advantage over single-agent therapy. The use of newer methods of drug administration such as intra-arterial therapy remains investigational, particularly as drug toxicity seems to increase.

ASTROCYTOMAS

The mainstay of treatment for grade 1 tumours is surgery, although there is debate about the value of surgery. It should be reserved for patients who are likely to improve in terms of their symptoms. Radiotherapy is used in selected patients and usually at the time of disease progression. Chemotherapy is not used unless there is a recurrence and the tumour grades transform to a higher-grade level. A large meta-analysis of randomised controlled trials has shown that in high-grade astrocytomas the addition of chemotherapy to radiotherapy does increase survival (Fine et al 1993).

OLIGODENDROGLIOMAS

Surgery remains the choice of treatment for these tumours, which tend to be slow growing. In tumours that are not resectable or which are aggressive, chemotherapy is considered. The use of radiotherapy is controversial. PCV regimens given in the adjuvant setting before radiotherapy have given good responses of over 70% in patients with aggressive tumours.

CNS LYMPHOMA

There is a high incidence of primary CNS lymphoma in patients with AIDS and it can occur at any age. The mainstay of treatment is chemotherapy followed by radiotherapy. The use of methotrexate-containing regimens, such as MACOP-B, can give a median survival of 3 years with combined radiotherapy use (Rampling 2002).

Gliomas: case 1

A 54-year-old man presented with a history of memory impairment. He had become increasingly more forgetful and his wife had noticed that his concentration appeared to be poor. Over the preceding weeks he had had increasing early morning headaches and his symptoms were worrying enough for his GP to arrange an urgent neurological referral. The neurologist arranged an urgent MRI scan of his brain and a large parieto-occipital tumour was found, with considerable surrounding oedema. He was put onto dexamethasone to alleviate his symptoms. The appearance of his tumour was considered highly suspicious for cancer and in view of his worsening condition the decision was made for him to undergo craniotomy and surgical debulking. The histology

continued on page 108

Gliomas: case 1 *continued*

confirmed this as a (WHO) grade IV glioblastoma multiforme of the right parieto-occipital lobe. He subsequently underwent radical radiotherapy but 7 months later his clinical condition worsened with falls, gait disturbance and confusion. Another MRI scan was done, which confirmed progressive disease at the original site as well as involvement of the contralateral hemisphere. Given the location and extent of disease it was felt that a surgical intervention would not be beneficial and that he should be referred to a medical oncologist for second-line treatment. He responded to a course of dexamethasone to regain his cognitive function and the two options offered for treatment were with either PCV or temozolamide. He opted for treatment with temozolamide.

Comments

This man has a high-grade, poorly differentiated tumour and his outlook remains poor. Surgery and postoperative radiotherapy are the mainstays of treatment. The median survival for these high-grade tumours remains at less than 1 year. The advantage of temozolamide is that it is given orally. It is indicated in recurrent anaplastic astrocytomas and glioblastoma multiforme. It is given at a dose of 200 mg/m^2 orally daily for 5 days and a reduced dose by 25% if patients have previously received chemotherapy. The toxicities with this treatment include grade 3 emesis, grade 2 myelosuppression and grade 1 alopecia. Phase II studies such as performed by EORTC (van den Bent et al 2003) have shown that the median time to progression can be delayed by 3 months in patients who are chemotherapy naïve.

HEAD AND NECK CANCERS

In the UK there are around 8000 cases of head and neck cancers with a worldwide incidence of 600 000 cases of head and neck cancers. Oral squamous cell carcinoma is the most common tumour of the oral cavity, affecting the oropharynx, particularly the palatine tonsils, and the base of tongue. An association has been found between the consumption of alcohol and smoking and molecular changes such as p53 mutations. The Epstein–Barr virus and the human papilloma virus have also been implicated. Most of these cancers occur in men over the age of 50 years of age.

The site of the primary tumour can lead to severe distress and morbidity in view of the effect on speech and nutrition. Typical presentations include pain, ulcers, epistaxis, cranial neuropathies and cervical lymphadenopathy. Advances in surgical techniques and the preservation of organ function have helped shape management of what can be a distressing and debilitating cancer. The development of the use of hyperfractionation of postoperative radiotherapy delivery, whereby small pulses of radiotherapy are given two or three times daily, helps to reduce toxicity of treatment and help local control.

The TNM staging (Vokes 1993) defines the findings of the presence of tumour as determined by clinical examination, endoscopy and imaging and has been updated to allow for tumour size specific for the primary site (Table 5.7).

TABLE 5.7 TNM staging for head and neck cancers

Grade	Description
Tumour (T)	
T0	No primary tumour
Tis	Carcinoma in-situ
T1	Tumour ≤ 2 cm
T2	Tumour > 2 cm and ≤ 4 cm
T3	Tumour > 4 cm
T4	Invasion of adjacent structures, e.g. tongue muscle
Lymph nodes (N)	
Nx	Regional lymph nodes cannot be assessed
N0	No regional lymph-node metastases
N1	Metastases to a single ipsilateral lymph node ≤ 3 cm
N2	Metastases to single ipsilateral lymph node (> 3 cm, ≤ 6 cm), multiple ipsilateral lymph nodes (none > 6 cm) or bilateral or contralateral lymph nodes (none > 6 cm)
N2a	Metastases to single ipsilateral lymph node (> 3 cm and ≤ 6 cm)
N2b	Metastases to multiple ipsilateral lymph nodes (none > 6 cm)
N2c	Metastases to a lymph node > 6 cm
N3	Metastases to a lymph node > 6 cm
Metastasis (M)	
M0	No evidence of distant metastases
M1	Distant metastases
Stage	
0	Tis, N0, M0
I	T1, N0, M0
II	T2, N0, M0
III	T3, N0, M0, T1–3, N1, M0
IV	T4, N0–1, M0 Any T, N2–3, M0 Any T and N, M1

Treatment is tailored to the site of the tumour. Most of these tumours are squamous cell cancers and loco-regional recurrence of tumour is common. Thus tumours of the oral cavity are considered for surgery, if resectable, followed by postoperative adjuvant radiotherapy. Patients with tumours of the hypopharynx and pyriform sinus are given concurrent chemotherapy and radiotherapy, and prognosis is likely to be poor in the latter group. In tumours of the larynx, the simultaneous use of chemotherapy and radiotherapy is considered.

Overall 30% of patients present with T1 and T2 lesions. The mainstay of treatment in the management of early-stage disease is single-modality treatment depending on the site of involvement or the combination of surgery and radiotherapy, the aim being curative. The type of treatment varies by the site and extent of regional disease, particularly nodal involvement. Radiotherapy has been associated with a better quality of life. Patients with stage I and stage II are curable usually undergoing surgery or radiotherapy, with up to 90% of patients being free of disease for at least 2 years.

In patients with more advanced disease, i.e. stage III or stage IV disease, surgery and radiotherapy may only cure 30% of patients and there is a high rate of locally recurrent disease. Chemotherapy is the mainstay of treatment. Toxicity of treatment is an important facet of treatment directed to prevent loco-regional disease recurrence.

Palliation is important in patients with advanced disease because the tumour can result in pain, dysphagia, speech dysfunction and neuropathies. The use of chemotherapy is considered in the palliative treatment of metastatic or recurrent disease. Response rates (defined as a reduction of at least 50% in the size of a tumour lasting for more than 1 month) have been low with single agents and the effect may only be for around 6 months at the most.

Chemotherapy single agents that are considered to be active in this group of patients include methotrexate, cisplatin, infusional 5-FU, docetaxel and paclitaxel; methotrexate and cisplatin are considered as standard chemotherapy. Patients more likely to respond are those who have small tumour bulk, good performance status and the least amount of previous treatment. Response rates can be as low as 10%, with median survival rates of 5 months in patients given methotrexate at standard doses. High-dose methotrexate simply leads to greater toxicity and is not recommended. Single-dose cisplatin can give response rates as high as 30% and, in some studies, has shown superior activity compared to methotrexate. Results of trials with paclitaxel and docetaxel have been encouraging.

Combination treatment with cisplatin and infusional 5-FU give a better response rate, even as high as 80%, although survival rates do not increase. This combination is considered the most active. Response rates are better if this combination is used in the neoadjuvant setting, with response rates exceeding 80%. However, no survival advantage is conferred using either adjuvant or neoadjuvant chemotherapy. The combination of cisplatin and methotrexate has not been shown to be superior to cisplatin or methotrexate alone. Although trials have recently looked at the newer drugs, such as the taxanes in combination with other agents, no survival advantage has been reached.

In patients with locally advanced tumour, which includes T3, T4, N1–N3 and M0 the use of neoadjuvant chemotherapy such as the use of cisplatin and 5-FU combinations, followed by surgery alone or surgery and radiotherapy, has been well studied. This treatment can lead to high response rates and complete response rates as high as 60% have been reached. However, survival rates have been disappointingly low (40% or less).

Concomitant chemotherapy in combination with radiotherapy has been investigated in randomised trials. The principle here is to use the chemotherapy agent as a radiosensitiser. Drugs such as cisplatin, bleomycin and mitomycin-C have been used. Although overall survival was reported as better with improvement in local control, there was an increase in toxicity (El-Sayed & Nelson 1996).

HEPATOCELLULAR CANCER

The rising incidence of hepatocellular cancer (HCC) reflects the latency between persistent hepatitis B infection (accounting for more than 50% of cases) and hepatitis C infection, haemachromatosis, alcohol consumption and aflatoxin exposure (fungal toxins) and the development of cirrhosis (Hall & Wild 2003). Worldwide it affects half a million people and the 5-year mortality is over 95%. The key to prevention is hepatitis B vaccination.

If hepatocellular cancer is localised, with no local spread, then it is potentially curative. The problem with this tumour is that the extent of the surgical resection is limited due to the presence of a likely cirrhotic liver. Transarterial catheter embolisation, ethanol injection, microwave coagulation and partial hepatectomy have been used to treat these patients. The problem, however, is the high intrahepatic recurrence rates with a 5-year survival less than 30%. Therefore, orthoptic liver transplantation is the only radical treatment to remove HCC and cirrhotic livers due to viral infections. This has been a controversial mode of treatment. Recurrence rates are high after liver resection or transplantation and 50% of patients have an aggressive cancer at the onset.

The role of chemotherapy is limited and a large proportion of hepatocellular cancers demonstrate resistance to chemotherapy agents with response rates even with combination therapy as low as 10%.

Mathurin (2003) performed a meta-analysis to evaluate adjuvant modalities after curative resection for hepatocellular carcinoma using randomised and non-randomised controlled trials. Four types of treatment were considered: preoperative transarterial chemotherapy, postoperative transarterial chemotherapy, systemic chemotherapy and a combination of systemic and transarterial chemotherapy. The conclusion called for new randomised controlled trials to evaluate postoperative transarterial chemotherapy, which was shown to improve survival and reduce recurrence rate.

Mathurin (1998) has also looked at the roles of doxorubicin, 5-FU, percutaneous ethanol injection, transarterial chemotherapy, the combination of Lipiodol with transarterial chemotherapy, tamoxifen and biological therapies such as interferon-α in the treatment of unresectable hepatocellular cancer. There was no significant survival benefit for any of the chemotherapy agents, with perhaps a small effect with tamoxifen and interferon-α. However, the variation in the number of relevant randomised trials, outcome measurements, study designs and treatments made it difficult to reach any meaningful conclusions. It may be that combination therapy with subcutaneous interferon-α and intra-arterial 5-FU, for example, shows some promise but further work is necessary to demonstrate a true survival benefit.

HODGKIN'S LYMPHOMA

The WHO classification of Hodgkin's disease is as follows:
Nodular lymphocyte-predominant Hodgkin's lymphoma (5% of cases).
Classical Hodgkin's lymphoma (95%):

- nodular sclerosis
- mixed cellularity classical Hodgkin's lymphoma
- lymphocyte-rich classical Hodgkin's lymphoma
- lymphocyte-depleted classical Hodgkin's lymphoma.

In the UK the incidence of Hodgkin's disease is around 1500 new cases per year, and a large proportion of these have a high chance of cure. The Reed–Steinberg cell is pathognomic of Hodgkin's disease, which is a rare cancer. The phenotype of the cancer is determined by immunoglobulin and lymphocytic analysis, the malignant cell originates from a B lymphocyte.

Most patients present with a painless neck lump, usually in the lower neck or supraclavicular area, systemic symptoms including night sweats, cough and breathlessness associated with mediastinal masses seen on chest X-ray, pruritus and fever and night sweats. There is classically a bimodal age of presentation.

CT scan is the main staging tool used and staging is defined by the Ann Arbor system, which has been modified to take into account the fact that laparotomy and splenectomy are no longer done to define the stage (Table 5.8).

Prognostic indices are used to determine predicted response to treatment and there are indices for localised and advanced disease based on analysis of patients with Hodgkin's disease. These include the stage, the age, the area involved, the ESR and the mediastinal/thoracic ratio (EORTC 1999).

TABLE 5.8 The Ann Arbor staging system for Hodgkin's lymphoma (from Lister 1989)

Stage	Description
I	Involvement of one lymph-node region or structure (e.g. spleen, thymus)
II	Two or more lymph-node regions on same side of diaphragm
III	Lymph nodes on both sides of diaphragm III1; with splenic hilar, coeliac or portal nodes III2: with para-aortic, iliac or mesenteric nodes
IV	Involvement of extragonadal site(s) beyond that designated E
Modifying features	
A	No symptoms
B	Fever, drenching night sweats, weight loss greater than 10% in 6 months
X	Bulky disease: greater than a third widening of the mediastinum Greater than 10 cm maximum diameter of nodal mass
E	Involvement of single, contiguous or proximal extra nodal site

TREATMENT OF LYMPHOCYTE-PREDOMINANT HODGKIN'S LYMPHOMA

The 5% of lymphocyte-predominant Hodgkin's lymphomas are treated as follows:

- Local disease, i.e. stages I and II: surgical excision and localised radiotherapy. There is a 94–98%, 8-year disease-specific survival.
- Advanced disease: treated as classical Hodgkin's disease.

TREATMENT OF CLASSICAL HODGKIN'S DISEASE

Localised disease

In the UK, this is defined as disease that is 2A or less. Between 20% and 30% of patients may relapse after radiotherapy alone. The combination of chemotherapy with radiotherapy may lower this relapse rate but survival may not be affected. The advantage of this combination is that the number of courses of chemotherapy and the amount of radiotherapy given to the patient may be reduced (Specht l998) and reduce the risk of secondary malignancies. The standard regimen is the ABVD regimen (doxorubicin, bleomycin, vinblastine and dacarbazine) given as a three-cycle course with a restricted involved radiotherapy field. Cure rates as high as 90% can be achieved.

Advanced disease

The role of radiotherapy in advanced disease is limited and makes no difference to overall survival. Chemotherapy is the mainstay of treatment in this group (Loeffler et al 1998). The ABVD is the standard treatment of choice (Canellos et al 1992). It compares to the original MOPP regimen, which was used initially in the treatment of advanced lymphoma. The advantage is less chance of infertility and secondary malignancies such as leukaemia. Toxicities of treatment include myelosuppression, emesis, respiratory and cardiotoxicity and neuropathy. Cure rates are around 70%.

Hodgkin's disease: case 1

A 66-year-old man presented to his GP with an 8-week history of a painless swelling in the neck. There was no other adenopathy apart from a bull neck with obvious bilateral lymphadenopathy. There was a history of weight loss of 2.5 kg in the past 6 weeks. There were no night sweats or pruritus. He underwent a cervical node biopsy, which confirmed a mixed cellularity Hodgkin's lymphoma and CT scan confirmed this showing no disease below the diaphragm. He commenced treatment with ChlVPP-PABlOE. This consisted of oral prednisolone, oral procarbazine, oral chlorambucil, prophylactic allopurinol (to cover the possibility of tumour lysis), itraconazole and alternate day co-trimoxazole (to cover opportunistic infection). He felt unwell after chemotherapy and syndrome of inappropriate antidiuretic hormone (SIADH) was diagnosed, which responded to fluid restriction. At week 7 after commencing chemotherapy, the patient's neck mass had receded, although he required hospital admission for grade 4 myelosuppression with a WCC of 0.4. Filgrastim (recombinant human G-CSF therapy) was prescribed and a good recovery made. He managed to complete six courses of delayed chemotherapy with a CT scan after treatment showing complete remission.

Comment

A randomised trial was to compare the efficacy of 6 cycles of PABlOE (prednisolone, doxorubicin, bleomycin, vincristine (Oncovin®) and etoposide) with three cycles of PABlOE that alternate with three cycles of ChlVPP (chlorambucil, vinblastine, procarbazine and prednisolone) in patients with advanced Hodgkin's disease was coordinated by the British National Lymphoma Investigation, Central Lymphoma Group (2001). The results were as shown in Table 5.9.

The ChlVPP is usually a well-tolerated regimen that is relatively effective and has a better toxicity profile than MOPP (nitrogen mustard, Oncovin® (vincristine), prednisolone and procarbazine), which was the gold standard before variations such as ABVD superseded it and which are better tolerated.

TABLE 5.9 Results from the British National Lymphoma Investigation (2001)

	Complete remission (CR) rates (%)	Overall survival (at 3 years) (%)
ChIVPP/PABlOE	78	91
PABlOE	64	85

The ChlVPP alternating with the PABlOE regimen is used. The ChlVPP regimen (chlorambucil, vinblastine, procarbazine and prednisolone) appears to be less toxic than ABVD.

Escalated BEACOPP (bleomycin, etoposide, doxorubicin, cyclophosphamide, Oncovin® (vincristine), procarbazine and prednisolone) has been used, particularly in high-risk patients, as has the Stanford V regimen, which is a combination of seven drugs.

Relapsed disease

High-dose chemotherapy and autologous stem-cell transplantation is the mainstay of treatment in this group, particularly if patients are younger than 65 years of age and fail first-line chemotherapy. Standard-dose chemotherapy is used to reduce tumour bulk before treatment with a graft and can sometimes predict whether a patient is likely to benefit from a graft. Cure rates of 30% can be achieved. Allogenic transplantation requires further clinical trials with follow-up data to ascertain its advantage.

LUNG CANCER

There are over 30 000 cases of lung cancer in England and Wales. Non-small-cell lung cancer (NSCLC) accounts for 85% of cases of lung cancer and has a 5-year survival of 5%. Molecular genetic studies have shown that mutations in tumour suppressor genes are critical in the multistep development of progression of lung cancers with loss of cell cycle control. Smoking remains the main risk factor; the risk of developing cancer is 20 times that compared to non-smokers.

Treatment depends on the histology and stage of the disease as well as the performance status of the patient. Surgery may be indicated in early stage (I or II) disease.

TYPES OF LUNG CANCER

- Small cell lung cancers comprise 15% of lung malignancies.
- Non-small-cell lung cancers comprise of the following histological types:
  - squamous cell: accounts for 35% of non-small-cell cases

- adenocarcinoma
- large cell
- bronchoalveolar
- undifferentiated.

SMALL CELL LUNG CANCER

The mainstay of treatment for this cancer is chemotherapy because it is considered to be a chemosensitive systemic disease with early metastatic disease. It is associated with paraneoplastic syndromes, including SIADH leading to hyponatraemia, Cushing's syndrome with ectopic ACTH secretion and Lambert–Eaton myasthenic syndrome.

Staging of small cell lung cancer

Performance status defined by the Karnofsky score or the ECOG performance state gives important prognostic information in this group of patients. SCLC can be divided into limited or extensive stage disease. Limited stage usually implies that there is only one lung involved, with ipsilateral lymph nodes involvement. Extensive disease implies spread to the other lung with lymph nodes involvement or distant organ spread. At presentation over 60% have extensive disease at the time of diagnosis. Patients with extensive disease may have 2-year survival rates of less than 2%.

When diagnosis is made, 40% of patients may have limited disease within the thorax. The median survival of patients with this stage of disease treated with chemotherapy and radiotherapy and the prophylactic cranial irradiation in selected cases is 18–24 months. Without treatment median survival can be only 6–12 weeks.

Patients with extensive disease may have metastatic disease involving organs such as bone marrow, brain and liver. With combination chemotherapy, the median survival of these patients is 7–9 months. The current standard chemotherapy regimenn is etoposide plus cisplatin or carboplatin (Carney 2002).

Use of chemotherapy in small cell lung cancer

The best response to treatment for either limited or extensive disease appears to be combination chemotherapy and, in some instances, combination chemotherapy with thoracic radiotherapy. Although single-agent chemotherapy has been used (with response rates that vary from 12 to 50%) this does not translate into a meaningful effect on survival. Agents that have been used include: cyclophosphamide (12–23% response rate), doxorubicin (15–20%), epirubicin (50%), vincristine (40–50%), vindesine (20–30%), cisplatin (5–30%), carboplatin (10–20%), etoposide (20–50%), paclitaxel (30%), docetaxel (20%), irinotecan (40%), topotecan (40%) and gemcitabine (27%).

Selected patients with limited disease who receive combination therapy can do well, with response rates averaging 90% (Potter 2002). The standard chemotherapy regimens used in the UK include:

- ACE (doxorubicin, cyclophosphamide and etoposide): this is used in both limited and extensive SCLC. It can give response rates of up to 80% with 40–65% complete response rates (Dearnley et al 2002). The median survival for limited-stage disease is 14 months and 9 months for extensive-stage disease. Toxicities include myelosuppression, cardiotoxicity and alopecia.
- Carboplatin–etoposide: used for both limited and extensive disease. There have been reports of 80% response rates with up to 15% complete response rates and a median survival of up to 12 months. Toxicities include myelosuppression, nephrotoxicity and ototoxicity.

Newer drug combinations, such as irinotecan and cisplatin, used in extensive SCLC have been encouraging, with an increase in median survival times compared to cisplatin and etoposide. However, despite these encouraging results, a significant number of patients may relapse (up to 80%). In patients with limited-stage SCLC the use of thoracic radiotherapy with chemotherapy has been shown to give a 5% increase in overall survival at 3 years compared with chemotherapy alone. Toxicity is increased, with the risk of damage to the lungs, oesophagus and bone marrow. Similarly, the use of prophylactic cranial irradiation has been shown to have a small impact on survival with a reduction in the risk of brain metastases. This is offset by a degree of cognitive impairment following irradiation. Oral etoposide has been used in patients who need salvage therapy in recurrent disease and who cannot tolerate combination chemotherapy. In untreated patients there is a 10% complete response rate with 85% response rate, which compares with 12% and less than 50% in previously treated patients.

NON-SMALL-CELL LUNG CANCER

The TNM system (American Joint Committee on Cancer (AJCC) staging of NSCLC is shown in Table 5.10. The staging system in terms of staging groups for NSCLC is shown in Table 5.11.

Surgery is recommended for stage I and II cancers. However, only one-third of patients are operable and those who have resected tumours have a 5-year survival rate of up to 40%. Standard chemotherapy for the purpose of palliation only is given in up to 20% of patients with advanced disease, with a median survival of 6–10 months if patients have stage IIIB or IV disease.

Chemotherapy trials have looked at the role of neoadjuvant chemotherapy in stage IIIA tumours. Little improvement in survival times has been found, but trials are ongoing. In the adjuvant setting, the Non-small-cell Lung Cancer Collaborative Group (1995) undertook a meta-analysis of trials with patients undergoing surgery and then receiving cisplatin-based combination therapy. They demonstrated a 5% survival benefit at 5 years in a selected

TABLE 5.10 TNM system (AJCC) staging of non-small-cell lung cancer

Grade	Description
Tumour (T)	
Tis	Carcinoma in situ with no invasion
T1	Tumour is less than 3 cm with no spread to the pleura with no lobar bronchi involvement
T2	Tumour is larger than 3 cm or involves a main bronchus but 2 cm distal from the carini or involvement of the visceral pleura or evidence of atelectasis without collapse
T3	Direct invasion and spread to the diaphragm or mediastinal pleura or parietal pericardium or involvement of the main bronchus less than 2 cm from the carini. Or collapse or a pneumonic process of the whole lung
T4	Invasion to oesophagus, trachea, great vessels, bone or pleural or pericardial effusions, or ipsilateral tumour nodules within lobe of the lung
Lymph nodes (N)	
N0	No spread to lymph nodes
N1	Ipsilateral peribronchial or hilar lymph nodes and intrapulmonary nodes
N2	Ipsilateral mediastinal or subcarinal nodes
N3	Contralateral mediastinal, hilar nodes or ipsilateral or contralateral scalene or supraclavicular lymph nodes
Metastasis (M)	
M0	No distant metastases
M1	Distant metastases

TABLE 5.11 Staging of non-small-cell lung cancer

Stage	Groups		
Stage 0	Tis	N0	M0
Stage IA	T1	N0	M0
Stage IB	T2	N0	M0
Stage IIA	T1	N1	M0
Stage IIB	T2	N1	M0
	T3	N0	M0
Stage IIIA	T1	N2	M0
	T2	N2	M0
	T3	N1	M0
	T3	N2	M0
Stage IIIB	Any T	N3	M0
	T4	Any N	M0
Stage IV	Any T	Any N	M1

group of patients. The same groups have demonstrated the advantage of using chemotherapy with radical radiotherapy in terms of a small increase in survival. This particularly applies to locally advanced unresectable stage III cancers. However, further studies are necessary to define optimal treatment (Potter 2002).

Lung cancer: case 1

A 61-year-old man presented to his GP with a 3-month history of back pain, loss of power in his legs and constipation. Spinal cord compression was suspected and he was urgently admitted into the nearest district general hospital. This was confirmed by MRI scan and a spinal decompression of a mass at the level of T8/T9 was performed. Biopsy of the mass showed it to be an adenocarcinoma and subsequent CT scan of the left lung confirmed the primary in the left upper lobe. Bone scan confirmed another metastatic lesion at the level of T5 and he underwent radiotherapy to his thoracic spine. Soon after completion of radiotherapy a palpable 2×3 lymph node was found in the left axilla. He was referred to a medical oncologist for consideration of palliative chemotherapy and with a performance status of 2 it was felt that carboplatin and vinorelbine would be a good option. Treatment was tolerated well and after four courses the disease was stable. The main toxicities of treatment were neutropenia and peripheral neuropathy with tingling of the fingertips.

Comment

This man has stage IV metastatic NSCLC. The aim of treatment here is palliation and the case highlights the combined modalities of radiotherapy and chemotherapy to achieve this. Meta-analysis of randomised controlled trials has shown that in advanced metastatic disease, platinum-based chemotherapy provides a survival benefit compared with best supportive care. New agents such as the taxanes, vinorelbine and gemcitabine have also shown benefit (Socinski 2004) and these beneficial effects have been confirmed through meta-analysis.

Vinorelbine is an example of an antimicrotubule agent. It is used with cisplatin in the neoadjuvant setting in the treatment of NSCLC. In the palliative care setting it is used either singly (it is also used in the palliation of mesothelioma) or in combination with platinum agents to palliate in the management of NSCLC (O'Brien 2004). It is usually given as an i.v. infusion but can be given orally. As a single agent it is better than supportive care in stage III and IV NSCLC. In combination with cisplatin, it has been shown to have a response rate of around 30% and a median 9-month survival time. Toxicity of treatment includes emesis, alopecia, myelosuppression, nephrotoxicity, neurotoxicity and phlebitis at the injection site. The combination of carboplatin with vinorelbine has been demonstrated to be a well-tolerated regimen in terms of toxicity. With this combination, a median progression-free period of 5.1 months has been demonstrated (O'Brien 2004).

The types of regimenns given in advanced disease include: MIC (mitomycin, ifosfamide and cisplatin) and MVP (mitomycin, videsine or vinblastine, and cisplatin). These patients are also at risk of renal toxicity from cisplatin-based chemotherapy. The purpose of chemotherapy here is palliation. There is debate about the best type of chemotherapy agent to use. Response rates remain low with 1-year survival rates of less than 40%. Chemotherapy should be offered only if there is a good performance status and there does not appear to be a superior combination regimen available. New agents such as taxanes, gemcitabine and vinorelbine used in combination with platinum agents provide equivalent survival improvement, as evident from randomised controlled trials, and seem to be well tolerated. The combination of carboplatin and paclitaxel produces a similar response and overall survival with a more favourable toxicity than cisplatin. Less than 5% of patients with NSCLC are alive at 5 years from diagnosis.

NICE-recommended drugs

- Docetaxel: indicated as second-line treatment of patients with locally advanced or metastatic NSCLC relapsing after prior chemotherapy.
- Paclitaxel: indicated in combination with cisplatin in patients who are not eligible for curative surgery or radiotherapy.
- Gemcitabine: licensed as first-line treatment for patients with locally advanced inoperable stage IIIA or IIIB or metastatic, stage IV, disease as either on its own or in combination with cisplatin.
- Vinorelbine: indicated as first-line treatment in patients with stage III or IV NSCLC, as monotherapy or in combination with other agents.

MESOTHELIOMA

There is a direct link between asbestos exposure and mesothelioma, which is a slow-growing tumour. The incidence of mesothelioma is expected to rise over the next 10 years and there could be close to 2500 deaths per year. The prognosis for this disease is poor and can be as low as 8 months.

Cisplatin is the most active agent used in the treatment of pleural mesothelioma. Combination treatment with cisplatin and doxorubicin has a response rate of around 28%. However, the issue is whether quality of life is increased by giving chemotherapy and studies are in progress to address this. The role of surgery and radiotherapy is limited.

MELANOMA AND NON-MELANOMA

MELANOMA

The incidence of melanoma (a malignant condition affecting the melanocytes) has increased over the past 20 years and it now accounts for 5000 deaths per year. The risk factors for melanoma include a history of sun exposure, family history of melanoma with germ-line mutations identified, the type of skin (e.g. atypical mole syndrome with four or more large naevi) and previous history of melanoma. The clinical features of a changing mole that might identify it as a melanoma include asymmetry, border irregularity, colour variation and diameter greater than 6 mm (Spicer & Gore 2002). Types of melanoma include the superficial spreading melanoma on the skin's surface, which is the most common, accounting for around 65–70%; nodular melanoma, lentigo maligna melanoma and acral melanoma, which occurs on the palms, soles or under nails.

Staging of melanoma

The new melanoma staging system from the American Joint Committee on Cancer (AJCC) uses the primary tumour (T), metastatic nodes (N) and distant metastases (M) system to match prognostic features of the primary and metastatic melanoma with survival outcome (Table 5.12). It includes melanoma thickness and ulceration, the number of metastatic lymph nodes and nodal metastases, which are classified as microscopic versus macroscopic. The M system uses the site of distant metastases and the presence of elevated serum lactic dehydrogenase. The presence of ulceration upstages patients with stage I, II and III disease. Clinical and pathological staging will take into account the staging information gained from an assessment of lymph node involvement such as using sentinel node biopsy (Balch 2001). In the presence of a tumour, a full-thickness biopsy is essential to make an accurate assessment. The Breslow system is used as a measure of tumour thickness. Sentinel node biopsy – the use of an intradermal blue dye injection with radiolabelled colloid – follows the path of the lymphatic channels to the first primary site-draining node, the sentinel node. This allows for an assessment of metastatic spread.

Treatment

Wide excision surgery is the treatment of choice in patients with localised disease with, if necessary, lymph node dissection. This has also been used to resect isolated visceral metastases.

The use of adjuvant therapy has largely been restricted to stage III disease in patients who are at risk of relapse, particularly with nodal involvement (Spicer & Gore 2002). The use of cytotoxic chemotherapy has not been shown to confer any significant improvement in survival. There have been adjuvant trials in the use of interferon-α. High-dose interferon has been used in some centres but there is debate about its effectiveness and toxicity associated with it in the adjuvant setting. Similarly, the role of vaccines is currently being evaluated.

TABLE 5.12 AJCC TNM staging for melanoma

Grade		Description
Tumour (T)	T1a	Melanoma in papillary dermis (Clark's level II) or melanoma filling the papillary dermis (Clark's level III), Breslow ≤ 1 mm thick, no ulceration
	T1b	Melanoma in the reticular dermis or melanoma in the subcutis (Clark's IV or V), Breslow ≤ 1 mm thick, or ulceration
	T2a	Breslow > 1 mm to ≤ 2 mm thick, no ulceration
	T2b	Breslow > 1 mm to ≤ 2 mm thick, ulceration
	T3a	Breslow > 2 mm to ≤ 4 mm thick, no ulceration
	T3b	Breslow > 2 mm to ≤ 4 mm thick, ulceration
	T4a	Breslow > 4 mm thick, no ulceration
	T4b	Breslow > 4 mm thick, ulceration
Lymph nodes (N)	N1	One node
	N1a	Microscopic
	N1b	Macroscopic
	N2	2–3 nodes or satellites without nodes
	N2a	Microscopic 2–3 nodes
	N2b	Macroscopic 2–3 nodes
	N2c	Satellites without nodes
	N3	More than 4 nodes
Metastasis (M)	M1a	Distant disease, e.g. skin, lymph node. Normal LDH
	M1b	Normal LDH with lung metastases
	M1c	Raised LDH with visceral metastases
Stage	IA	T1a, N0, M0
	IB	T1b or 2a, N0, M0
	IIA	T2b or T3a, N0, M0
	IIB	T3b or 4a, N0, M0
	IIC	T4b, N0, M0
	IIIA	Any Ta, N1a or N2a, M0
	IIIC	Any Tb, N1b, N2b, M0 Any T, N3, M0
	IV	Any T, any N, M1a Any T, any N, M1b Any T, any N, M1c

LDH, lactate dehydrogenase. Stage IA has a 10-year survival of 90%; whereas stage IV < 20%.

The overall median survival of patients with systemic metastasis from melanoma is about 6 months. Patients with non-visceral metastases at first relapse, i.e. in skin, subcutaneous tissues, distant lymph nodes and lung, have a better survival rate than patients with visceral (liver, bone, brain) metastases (Lee 1995). In recurrent or metastatic disease, surgery may be used for single-site recurrences whereas radiotherapy is used as palliation for metastatic disease. The role of chemotherapy and immunotherapy in metastatic disease has been limited, with dacarbazine being the single agent with the best response rate of up to 20% and duration of response of up to 10 months. There is no advantage in the use of combination chemotherapy that includes the addition of immunotherapy. The main side effect of dacarbazine is emesis, which can be controlled through the use of $5-HT_3$ receptor antagonists.

NON-MELANOMA

Basal cell carcinoma

Surgery is the treatment of choice. The mainstay of drug treatment is with topical 5-FU. The usual type of BCC treated in this way is the thin BCC rather than the deep-rooted BCC. The treatment involves 25% concentrations of topical 5-FU in petrolatum under occlusion for 3 weeks using daily dressings; 5-year recurrence rates of around 20% have been reported, with good cosmetic results.

Other types of treatment include interferon-2α and interferon-2β, with complete response rates of around 60%. Side effects of treatment include fever and malaise. Topical imiquimod has been used; this is a cytokine and interferon inducer. Side effects of treatment include local skin reactions. Other non-drug treatment includes radiotherapy and cryotherapy.

Squamous cell cancer

The mainstay of treatment is surgery or radiotherapy. These cancers can recur or metastasise in less than 10% of patients; this is influenced by the tumour size and depth. Metastatic disease can be treated using drugs, although with varying degrees of success, and there is a poor outlook with 10-year survival rates that can be less than 10%. The drugs used include bleomycin, methotrexate, vincristine, 5-FU and hydroxyurea. Combinations of cisplatin, 5-FU and bleomycin have shown some complete remissions.

MULTIPLE MYELOMA

In the UK the incidence of myeloma is 2500 cases per year, most patients being over the age of 60 years. Multiple myeloma is a malignant disease of plasma cells. The effect of this is an accumulation of plasma cells that can lead to bone marrow infiltration resulting in anaemia, increased risk of infections, lytic bone lesions and hypercalcaemia. Plasma cell leukaemia reflects a high absolute plasma cell burden within the marrow plasma cells. Other complications include renal failure, bone pain with the risk of pathological fractures and vertebral body collapse, and spinal cord compression. However, patients may be asymptomatic and a raised ESR may be an early indicator of disease activity.

The diagnosis is usually made based on serum and urine immunoelectrophoresis looking for a paraprotein and Bence Jones protein in urine. Bone marrow aspirate and trephine biopsy and skeletal survey confirm diagnosis and the extent of disease. β2-microglobulin is measured and used as a prognostic factor, as is loss of the Rb gene on chromosome 13, which occurs in one-third of cases. The median overall survival is up to 7 years and the complete remission rate is as high as 60%, with the median event-free survival being 24–43 months.

Monoclonal gammopathy of unknown origin may be a premyelomatous condition that, over time, transforms into myeloma in 20% of patients over 20 years. These patients should have their paraprotein levels measured regularly, i.e. 3- to 6-monthly and should be kept under surveillance for signs of active disease. Those patients who are classified as being between monoclonal gammopathy of unknown origin and myeloma are known as patients with smouldering myeloma.

Currently, the staging system for myeloma is being revised to take into account prognostic factors such as β2-microglobulin. However, the Durie–Salmon staging system has been used historically (Table 5.13). The survival rates based on stage indicate a 5-year survival of about:

- 50% for stage I
- 40% for stage II
- 10–25% for stage III disease.

TABLE 5.13 Durie–Salmon staging system

Stage	Description
I	Represents low tumour volume disease with low monoclonal IgG and IgA levels, low levels of Bence Jones protein excretion in the urine, normal calcium levels or mildly raised and a haemoglobin > 10 g/dL and at most one lytic bone lesion
II	Medium tumour mass with parameters between stages I and III
III	Represents high tumour bulk with any of high levels of monoclonal Ig levels Further subdivisions depend on renal function such that stage A disease has a creatinine < 175 µmmol/L whereas stage B disease has a creatinine > 175 µmmol/L

TABLE 5.14 The new international staging system for multiple myeloma

Stage	Description
I	β2M < 3.5 mg/L and albumin ≥ 3.5 g/dL
II	β2M < 3.5 mg/L and albumin < 3.5 g/dL or β2M 3.5–5.5 mg/L
III	β2M > 5.5 mg/L

B2M is only reliable if the patient has normal renal function.

The new international staging system for multiple myeloma is simpler to use and has taken transplanted patients into account (Table 5.14).

The good risk groups are those with an age < 60 years. In patients aged > 60 years with a platelet count < 130 000/mm^2 and above normal LDH levels, survival is < 2 years.

The aim of treatment is to achieve a complete remission. Patients who do not are compromised in terms of quality of life and long-term survival. Treatment is reserved for stage IA patients by careful follow-up.

Complete remission is defined as (Sirohi & Powles 2004):

- at least 6 weeks of the absence of serum and urine monoclonal paraprotein
- less than 5% plasma cells in bone marrow aspirate and trephine biopsy
- no increase in the size or number of lytic bone lesions
- no soft tissue plasmacytomas.

Historically, the principle of treatment is induction therapy, followed by high-dose chemotherapy. The most common drugs used for induction therapy is the combination of melphalan and prednisolone (MP) giving response rates of up to 60%. The usual regimenn is 4 days of treatment every 4-6 weeks.

Other regimens that have been used have shown a better response rate but meta-analysis has confirmed that combination chemotherapy is no better in terms of survival (Myeloma Trialists' Collaborative Group 1998). The ABCM regimen (doxorubicin, BCNU, cyclophosphamide and melphalan), the VAD regimen (vincristine, doxorubicin and dexamethasone) and the CVAMP regimen (cyclophosphamide, vincristine, doxorubicin and methylprednisolone) are examples of combination chemotherapy agents that have been used in induction therapy. Regimens are used depending on whether stem-cell transplant is to be done, the age and renal function.

Relapse is likely to occur after induction therapy. The standard therapy now given is induction treatment followed by high-dose melphalan, i.e. 200 mg/m^2, with peripheral stem-cell rescue either as a single or possible double (tandem) autologous transplant. High-dose treatment leads to significantly better event-free survival and overall survival as shown by randomised trials (Child et al 2003). However, this does not lead to cure. The median survival is close to 7 years although all patients will relapse and it is possible to retreat relapsed patients with the same drug treatment given initially with a 50% response rate. Thalidomide and thalidomide analogues have been used in relapsed patients and have given response rates over 50%. The option of allogenic transplant is available but transplant-related mortality is high and the long-term overall survival beyond 5 years is only 35%.

In the management of myeloma, the potential complications of myeloma, such as hypercalcaemia, anaemia, renal failure, lytic bone lesions and pathological fractures, must also be considered. Bisphosphonates during treatment and for long-term maintenance help to prevent osteoporosis, bone pain and risk of fractures, and treat hypercalcaemia after hydration and the use of corticosteroids. They are recommended for all patients with myeloma. Radiotherapy is used to alleviate bone pain and as part of myeloablative treatment before transplantation in allogenic transplant.

Erythropoietin is used to treat anaemia during chemotherapy. Combination chemotherapy with vincristine, doxorubicin and dexamethasone is used to control renal failure when standard measures such as hydration and correction of metabolic disorders (Kyle & Arkoma 2004) and the use of plasmaphoresis and dexamethasone fails to correct an acute deterioration in renal function.

NEUROENDOCRINE TUMOURS

In the UK there may be up to 1500 new cases of neuroendocrine tumours each year. These can be classed into benign or malignant functional or non-functional tumours as below, and arise from neuroendocrine cells. There is an association with multiple endocrine neoplasia (MEN):

- Functional: carcinoid tumours, insulinomas, gastrinomas and glucagonomas. Carcinoid tumours typically present with wheeze, diarrhoea and flushing.
- Non-functional tumours: present as masses from respective organs.

The essence of treatment of these patients should be by multidisciplinary teams in a tertiary centre.

The drug treatment of choice for non-resectable symptomatic patients is the somatostatin analogues, which include lanreotide and octreotide. The somatostatin analogues can control hormone secretion and stabilise tumour growth by inhibiting peptide hormone release. This can result in symptomatic relief in up to 70% of patients and a similar biochemical response. Gastrointestinal side effects include nausea, cramps, diarrhoea and gallstones. Lanreotide is a long-acting analogue that acts over a 2–4-week period.

Chemotherapy may be used for palliation of neuroendocrine tumours, particularly in the presence of progressive disease. Streptozocin-based combinations, especially with doxorubicin, remain the first-line standard. Interferon has also been used; this acts to stimulate the immune system and control hormone secretion and tumour growth. Side effects include myalgia and headache with fever. It has been used in combination with infusional 5-FU.

Neuroendocrine tumours: case 1

A 57-year-old woman presented to her GP with a history of weakness, tiredness and nocturia. Blood tests were arranged and she was found to be profoundly hypokalaemic with potassium of 2.5 mmol/L. This led to an immediate hospital admission for intravenous potassium replacement.

She underwent a series of investigations to determine the cause of her hypokalaemia. She had a series of hormonal and endocrine tests, which indicated a raised C-peptide and insulin level. An islet cell tumour was suspected. A CT scan of the upper abdomen confirmed a mass in the head of the pancreas in the uncinate process. Laparoscopy showed no evidence of peritoneal disease and thus a formal abdominal incision was performed. This showed the mass extending to the superior mesenteric vessels. She thus underwent a pylorus preserving pancreaticoduodenectomy. Histology confirmed this as malignant tumour with five out of five lymph nodes containing metastatic tumour with clear resection margins. She was prescribed creon for steatorrhoea and was referred for an oncology opinion.

In view of the nature of the invasive disease, adjuvant chemotherapy with streptozocin and doxorubicin was offered. She had eight courses of treatment but a scan at the end of treatment revealed a significant increase in coeliac lymph nodes and liver metastases. She required readmission when the potassium level fell to 2 mmol/L and was found to be hyperglycaemic, with a raised cortisol > 1500 mmol/L and a raised serum ACTH at 300 mmol/L. Metryapone was commended, as was octreotide, and, together with fluids, potassium replacement and correction of the hyperglycaemia the patient made a good recovery. Second-line chemotherapy was commenced with carboplatin and capecitabine but after two courses of treatment there was progressive disease in the liver and treatment was stopped. The patient underwent a somatostatin receptor scintigraphy, which indicated low activity and it was felt that somatostatin-receptor-targeted therapy would not be an option. Experimental therapy may be considered.

Comment

This is an example of a neuroendocrine tumour, which is a rare tumour with an incidence of 1 in 100 000. It is characterised by the differentiation of stem cells into adult endocrine-secreting cells. The classification of these tumours is based on the hormones that they secrete, although they can be non-functional: insulinomas, gastrinomas, vipomas, somatostatinomas, pancreatic polypeptide. Thus symptoms are either through the effect of the hormone, local tumour spread or metastatic spread.

In this case it is likely that the tumour is producing a growth-hormone-secreting peptide. In islet-cell cancers the hormone that is predominantly present may change. The two most important prognostic factors are lymph node involvement and the size of the primary tumour. There was a need for chemotherapy postoperatively in view of metastatic spread.

continued on page 128

Neuroendocrine tumours: case 1 *continued*

As a single agent streptozocin has shown a good response rate at around 40–50%. Its main side effects are myelosuppression, renal impairment and nausea and vomiting. In combination with doxorubicin, response rates have been close to 70%. The median duration of response is around 12 months.

Somatostatin is a peptide that reduces levels of insulin, gastrin and glucagon. It also inhibits the release of growth hormone and the suppression of insulin and glucagon. The finding that somatostatin receptors are found on neuroendocrine tumour cells opens up the possibility of new treatment regimens. Octreotide is a somatostatin analogue that has been shown to have some activity in stabilising metastatic endocrine tumours such as glucagonoma, vipoma and gastrinoma. Its main side effects include gastrointestinal symptoms such as diarrhoea, gallstones and steatorrhoea. Interferon-α has also shown to have some activity.

Radiolabelled somatostatin analogues are used to help determine the presence of neuroendocrine tumours. They bind to the same sites as endogenous somatostatin, which makes them sensitive indicators of somatostatin-receptor-bearing neuroendocrine tumours. Treatment with radioactive labelled octreotide could then be possible.

Surgical resection is an option in single hepatic metastases, as is chemoembolisation for metastatic liver disease.

In this case, the secretion of ACTH could be representative of a multiple endocrine neoplasia (MEN) whereby there is a pituitary adenoma secreting ACTH. There is also an association with excess secretion of parathyroid hormone and hypercalcaemia. A pituitary MRI scan may be indicated.

Liver metastasis is the main organ involved in metastatic spread. Surgery to remove isolated hepatic metastases is possible. Hepatic arterial embolisation, radiofrequency ablation and cryosurgical techniques may also be useful in selected patients.

NON-HODGKIN'S LYMPHOMA

The incidence of non-Hodgkin's lymphoma (NHL) is rising. In adults it accounts for just fewer than 5% of cancers, whereas in childhood in Western countries it can account for up to 10% of cancer cases. The WHO classification of NHL reflects the heterogeneous nature of this cancer in terms of histological diagnosis and there has recently been a new classification called the REAL (Revised European–American Lymphoma) classification for NHL. This can be broadly divided into B-cell and T-cell/NK (natural killer) cell neoplasms. Of the B-cell lymphomas, the more common tend to be follicular lymphoma and diffuse large B-cell lymphoma. Other subtypes include

TABLE 5.15 Ann Arbor staging system for non-Hodgkin's lymphoma

Stage	Description
I	Single lymph-node region or single extra lymphatic organ
II	Two or more lymph-node sites affected on same side of diaphragm Disease may involve local extralymphatic site
III	Lymph-node regions affected on both sides of diaphragm with or without involvement of spleen or local lymphatic site
IV	Disseminated disease involving one or more extra lymphatic organs with or without lymph-node involvement

Burkitt's lymphoma, hairy cell leukaemia and mantle lymphomas. Of the T-cell neoplasms, mycosis fungoides and peripheral T-cell lymphoma are the most common histological types. The Ann Arbor staging system is used to stage the spread of disease (Table 5.15).

The importance of staging is to guide treatment and gain prognostic information. Investigations used to guide staging include clinical history assessing for B symptoms of systemic disease, clinical examination, haematological and biochemical profiles. Markers of disease include ESR, LDH, and serum β2-microglobulin. Chest X-ray, bone marrow and biopsy and CT scan of the abdomen, pelvis and abdomen are necessary to accurately define the stage of spread.

Cases of NHL are treated and curable with chemotherapy. Radiotherapy is used in the initial treatment of lymphomas. The two most common histological types are follicular and diffuse B-cell lymphoma.

FOLLICULAR LYMPHOMA

Most patients have stage III and IV disease but in those with stage I and II disease, involved field radiotherapy can give 5-year relapse-free survival rates of up to 80% and overall survival rates of up to 100%. Although single-agent and combination therapy have been used, there are varying reports about the effect on disease-free survival or overall survival.

In patients with advanced disease, i.e. stage III or stage IV, there is debate about the best treatment. These tumours tend to be indolent with median survival of 7–10 years.

Single-agent chlorambucil has been used and can give 5-year survival rates of up to 80% and an 8-year median survival time. Usual toxicities include mild myelosuppression and emesis and hair loss with the risk of secondary leukaemias. Combination treatment with CVP (cyclophosphamide, vincristine and prednisolone) shows similar survival times.

Toxicities are similar but more severe and include neurotoxicity.

NICE has approved rituximab, a monoclonal antibody for stage III or IV follicular lymphoma, if the disease is resistant or has relapsed. In Phase II trials there were response rates of 50% in low-grade lymphomas. Rituximab has been used in combination with CHOP (cyclophosphamide, vincristine, doxorubicin and prednisolone) as first-line and relapsed therapy of low-grade NHL, with response rates over 90%.

Gemcitabine has been used in pretreated patients with NHL and can give response rates as high as 70% with low-grade toxicity.

Fludarabine has been used as a single agent and has given response rates of around 60%. Its use is as a single or as part of combination therapy in third-line treatment of relapsed patients.

Non-Hodgkin's lymphoma: case 1

A 65-year-old woman had presented with a 2–3-month history of abdominal pain associated with 3.5 kg weight loss. An ill-defined mass was found in the central abdomen on ultrasound. She was found to have a raised CA-125 (cancer antigen 125), a raised LDH of 600 and abnormal liver function tests with a raised alkaline phosphatase of 400 and a raised ALT of 170. A subsequent CT scan showed a left central abdominal mass of 12 × 13 cm. The underlying structures were displaced and so it was difficult to see what the origin of the mass was. She underwent a trucut biopsy of her mesenteric mass and the mass was found to be high-grade B-cell non-Hodgkin's lymphoma. She was staged as IIIB and was put onto rituximab-CHOP chemotherapy. She completed eight courses of chemotherapy, CT scan after her fourth course showing significant disease regression, her main complications being neutropenia and anaemia, which required transfusion. Her liver function tests also reversed to normal, indicating probably lymphomatous infiltration at presentation. CT scan after her eighth course showed she was in complete remission.

Comments

CHOP in combination with rituximab has led to over 90% response rates in Phase II trials.

Rituximab (R) is a monoclonal antibody against the CD20 antigen. An example of how well it performs is evident from a multicentre Phase II trial of R-CHOP (Czuczman 2004) in patients with CD20-positive, low-grade, B-cell, non-Hodgkin's lymphoma. Some of these patients were newly diagnosed, others had relapsed; they received six courses of R-CHOP. Overall response rate was 100% with 87% of patients achieving a complete response or unconfirmed complete response. There was a good length of response duration lasting over 80 months.

DIFFUSE LARGE B-CELL LYMPHOMAS

These interesting lymphomas are aggressive tumours that account for the majority of NHL lymphomas. Although they are aggressive they are curable in 40% of cases. In stage I and II disease, the standard treatment is the use of a shortened course of chemotherapy, such as CHOP, followed by involved-field radiotherapy. Chemotherapy is given for intermediate and advanced disease (i.e. stage III and IV disease). The CHOP regimen is the standard course of therapy with long-term survival in up to 40% of patients treated. Pretreatment factors such as LDH levels and stage predict for outcome as do age, number of extranodal sites involved and performance status. Treatment is 3-weekly and cardiac monitoring is required with cumulative doses of doxorubicin to prevent cardiac toxicity. It requires antiemetic therapy and myelosuppressive treatment; hair loss is inevitable. Other side effects include neuropathy, haemorrhagic cystitis and subfertility. Rituximab is used as part of combination therapy with CHOP and has a better response rate than CHOP alone. It is recommended through NICE for stage II, III and IV disease as first-line combination therapy.

Other agents used include PMITCEBO (prednisolone, mitoxantrone (doxorubicin in place of mitoxantrone if necessary), cyclophosphamide, etoposide, bleomycin, vincristine plus methotrexates). This has similar response rates to CHOP. The toxicity profile is slightly less aggressive than CHOP.

Patients who relapse within 2 years of first-line therapy are considered for platinum based regimen to get complete response first and then considerations for high dose chemotherapy and peripheral autologous stem-cell harvesting.

OESOPHAGEAL CANCER

Worldwide, oesophageal cancer is the sixth leading cause of death from cancer. It accounts for 5% of all cancer deaths in the UK. Seventy-five per cent of all adenocarcinomas are found in the distal oesophagus, whereas squamous cell carcinomas are more evenly distributed between the middle and lower third. These two types of cancer account for 90% of all cancers of the oesophagus. At diagnosis, over 50% of patients may have unresectable tumours that are locally advanced or metastatic disease; these patients may require palliative treatment to relieve progressive dysphagia. The overall survival rate is less than 10% with a median survival of 9 months. A prognostic index may be used to determine how patients may progress (Chau 2004).

In patients with localised disease who are suitable, surgery remains the preferred option (Malthaner 2004). Surgery can be extensive and radical, e.g. total oesophagectomy with lymphadenectomy. However, even in this group 5-year survival may be around 25% at best. Surgery can be used for stage I disease when the tumour extends only as far as the lamina propria or the submucosa, stage II disease when it extends as far as the adventitia with possible regional node involvement or stage III disease when adjacent structures are involved, with or without regional node involvement. In an attempt to improve survival rates, clinical trials have looked at the role of neoadjuvant or adjuvant therapy, which includes the use of chemotherapy, radiotherapy or both.

Neoadjuvant chemotherapy (i.e. chemotherapy before surgery) using cisplatin and 5-FU has shown a small benefit in terms of survival benefit and 2-year survival rates of 30–40% with preoperative chemotherapy plus surgery have been reported (Medical Research Council Oesophageal Cancer Working Party 2002). Similarly, despite the widespread use of preoperative chemotherapy and radiotherapy, the survival benefits remain low. Meta-analyses of neoadjuvant trials have shown a degree of local control but no survival advantage for neoadjuvant chemotherapy or concurrent chemoradiotherapy. If patients receive neoadjuvant treatment and achieve a histologically confirmed complete response they do seem to have significant better survival (Richel & Vervenne 2004). Neoadjuvant chemoradiotherapy gives a higher rate of complete responses compared to neoadjuvant chemotherapy (30% versus 15%) but this is associated with increased morbidity (Fiorica et al 2004).

Symptoms in many patients with advanced (i.e. stage IV) disease with coeliac node, cervical node or distant metastases, can be helped by palliative chemotherapy. However, the response to chemotherapy typically lasts no

---

Oesophageal cancer: case I

A 65-year-old man presented with a history of weight loss and dysphagia for solids over a 2-month period. Upper GI endoscope revealed a lesion in the oesophagus which when biopsied confirmed as a poorly differentiating carcinoma. A CT scan indicated a liver metastasis. He was referred to a medical oncologist for consideration of chemotherapy. He was classified as having stage III tumour. A MUGA scan was performed in view of a consideration of anthracycline-type chemotherapy and this showed an impaired cardiac fraction of 47% with inferolateral hypokinesis. As the patient was not eligible for a clinical trial in view of his ejection fraction, he was commenced on carboplatin and capecitabine. His EDTA was normal. Two courses of treatment were completed. However, his condition deteriorated, his performance status fell to 3 and it was decided to withhold any further treatment apart from palliation of his symptoms.

Comments

This illustrates the importance of checking for cardiac disease when determining whether a patient should receive an anthracycline-based treatment, which in this case would have been epirubicin in the ECF regimen (epirubicin, cisplatin and 5-FU). The aim of treatment is clearly palliation but it was hoped that the combination of agents that are perhaps less toxic and better tolerated than cisplatin and intravenous 5-FU might be acceptable for this patient.

longer than a few months and survival beyond 1 year is unusual. The agents used include cisplatin, 5-FU and the anthracyclines such as epirubicin. Drugs such as the taxanes and irinotecan in combination with the platinum agents, e.g. cisplatin, are currently undergoing randomised trials and results have been encouraging. Other treatment options in dysphagia include self-expanding metal stent placements, brachytherapy with external beam radiation and dilatation.

OVARIAN CANCER

Ovarian cancer is the fifth leading cause of cancer death in European women and is the most common cause of death among women with a gynaecological malignancy. It is often diagnosed in advanced phase (stage III, IV). Prognosis is poor despite activity shown by chemotherapy agents. In the UK there are 6000 new cases and 4500 deaths from ovarian cancer. The overall 5-year survival rate is poor because patients present late; it can be as low as 30%. The most common type is the epithelial type.

There is a survival advantage in tumour debulking and the majority of patients get a full staging laparotomy, a total abdominal hysterectomy, bilateral salpingo-oophorectomy and omentectomy. Staging of tumour from histological samples is defined by the FIGO system, with 90% of ovarian cancers being of epithelial origin. Early-stage limited disease is defined as stage I disease. Stage IA patients with well-differentiated tumours have a 90% 5-year survival with surgery alone. However, in stage I disease there is a group of patients in whom the tumours may have breached the capsule, with washings and ascites containing malignant cells; these patients have a worse prognosis and are staged as IC. These patients and patients with grade 3 poorly differentiated tumours or clear-cell histology need adjuvant chemotherapy.

Two important trials have looked at the role of adjuvant chemotherapy:

- The ICON-I trial: randomised patients to platinum treatment either immediately after surgery or at relapse.
- The ACTION trial: randomised patients based on stage (from IA to II) and histology to either immediate chemotherapy or platinum-based treatment at relapse.

The data from both trials showed a significant survival benefit for those who received immediate treatment with a 7% absolute difference in overall survival at 5 years and a reduction in the risk of recurrence.

The standard first-line agent for ovarian cancer is carboplatin, which is better tolerated than cisplatin, and meta-analysis has shown that there is no difference in efficacy. It is usually given in combination with paclitaxel. Treatment is usually given on a 3-weekly schedule for a maximum of six cycles and this combination has been shown to be better tolerated than cisplatin combinations:

- Frail patients should receive carboplatin alone.
- 80% of cases achieve objective response with platinum-containing regimens.
- Over 20% of patients progress while receiving initial platinum-based treatment and are defined refractory to chemotherapy.
- 40% of patients relapse or progress within 12 months and 20% after 12 months from the end of first-line platinum chemotherapy.

Paclitaxel has a role as standard first-line treatment in combination with platinum compounds. NICE revised its guidance on the use of paclitaxel in the treatment of ovarian cancer in January 2003. It now recommends that paclitaxel in combinations with platinum-based compounds, or platinum-based therapy alone, are offered as alternatives for first-line chemotherapy.

Patients with stage II disease should receive surgical treatment followed by chemotherapy, whereas those with stage III disease need debulking surgery followed usually by six courses of chemotherapy. In stage II disease, 5-year survival can be as high as 50% whereas in stage III it is around 25%. Stage IV disease may be inoperable and chemotherapy is tailored to performance status, with 5-year survival rates of 10%. Chemotherapy has been used in this stage to lessen tumour bulk before surgery.

The time for treatment of relapsed disease depends on tumour bulk, residual tumour greater than 5 cm and the performance status of the patient. CA-125 is a sensitive tumour marker of relapse. Symptomatic patients with a rising CA-125 need treatment. Patients who do not secrete CA-125 need follow-up with regular scans. Patients who relapse within 6 months of chemotherapy are likely to have poor response to chemotherapy. Those who relapse after 6 months can be given platinum treatment and are more likely to respond. Second-line treatment includes drugs that are non-cross-resistant with platinum. Single-agent drugs used for patients who relapse within 6 months of platinum treatment include liposomal doxorubicin, paclitaxel, topotecan and chlorambucil. Response rates vary from 10 to 25%.

Liposomal encapsulation of anticancer drugs offers advance of increasing drug efficiency while decreasing toxicity. Pegylated liposomal doxorubicin (Caelyx®) is a formulation of doxorubicin encapsulated in small stealth liposomes. Its tissue distribution gives it a high concentration of active agent into tumour. Dose-limiting toxicities include hand–foot skin reactions and mucositis. In clinical trials, Caelyx® is associated with less cardiac toxicity and myelotoxicity.There have been responses to a broad range of tumours including ovarian cancer, hepatocellular and head and neck cancers.

Topotecan has been recommended by NICE in relapsed ovarian cancer. Chemotherapy for patients with bowel obstruction is favoured if it presents in patients who are chemotherapy naïve or there has been a long treatment-free

Ovarian cancer: case 1

A 65-year-old woman presented to her GP with postmenopausal bleeding. A subsequent ultrasound showed a 6-cm ovarian mass. A CA-125 was elevated at 90 u/mL. Referral to a gynaecological specialist in gynaecological malignancies led to an MRI scan that demonstrated a multicystic ovarian mass and no other abdominal or pelvic abnormalities. A total abdominal hysterectomy and bilateral salpingo-oophorectomy with peritoneal biopsy was performed. Subsequent histology confirmed a poorly differentiated serous carcinoma in the omentum and the peritoneum. This is classed as stage IIIb disease. She was referred to a cancer centre for consideration of chemotherapy. Carboplatin at an AUC 7 dose was commenced with Taxol® and gemcitabine as part of a study. After six courses of carboplatin her CA-125 had dropped to normal with a normal CT scan showing no evidence of recurrent disease. Her main side effects during chemotherapy had been fatigue and myelosuppression. However, on review 18 months later she had a recurrence on CT scan with a new peritoneal nodule. As she had gone over 1 year she was offered carboplatin as a repeat course. There would also be the opportunity to put her into a clinical trial of carboplatin together with a new experimental agent going through phase I trials. She completed her six courses of carboplatin and at present remains in remission.

Comments

CA-125 is a surface antigen that originates from papillary serous cystadenocarcinoma. It is detectable in the peritoneum, pleura and pericardium, and is used as a marker for ovarian cancer. It is best used when elevated as a response to treatment. It is seen in other malignancies, such as breast, cervix and colorectal cancers, as well as in non-malignant conditions such as fibroids, pregnancy and pancreatitis.

Staging for ovarian cancer is defined by the FIGO staging as follows:

- stage I: ovarian cancer is confined to the ovary or ovaries
- stage II: spread beyond the ovaries but confined to the pelvis (i.e. could be in the bladder, uterus or rectum)
- stage III: spread to the peritoneum ± lymph nodes
- stage IV: distant spread.

In this case, stage IIIB represents histological confirmed implants of abdominal peritoneal surfaces, none exceeding 2 cm in diameter with node-negative disease. The Calvert formula is used to calculate the dose of carboplatin in ovarian cancer (Professor Hilary Calvert is Professor of Medical Oncology at the University of Newcastle Upon Tyne). Carboplatin dosage is calculated from GFR (glomerular filtration rate, measured in mL/min) and target AUC (area under the curve, measured in mg/mL/min) of carboplatin:

$$\text{Carboplatin dosage (mg)} = \text{AUC} \times (\text{GFR} + 25)$$

continued on page 136

> **Ovarian cancer: case I** *continued*
>
> The target AUC (mg/mL/min) depends on whether carboplatin is given as combination chemotherapy. The aim is for an AUC of 6–8 mg/mL/min if carboplatin is the sole drug and there has been no previous treatment. Consider dose reduction aiming for an AUC of 4–6 mg/mL/min if carboplatin is being given as combination chemotherapy, e.g. with cyclophosphamide, or if previous treatment has been given.
>
> There have been trials in women with chemotherapy-naïve stage IC–IV ovarian cancer who have been treated with carboplatin, paclitaxel and gemcitabine (Harries 2004). Response rates of over 80% have been reported, with significant drops in CA-125. The median progression-free survival time has been close to 20 months. Toxicities include grade 3 or 4 neutropenia, breathlessness associated with interstitial chest X-ray changes, which reversed when treatment was completed.

interval. In these groups tumour response rates of over 50% have been reported relieving obstruction.

Paclitaxel is active in relapsed platinum-resistant ovarian cancer and well tolerated. Significant side effects other than alopecia are uncommon. In the early 1990s, paclitaxel became a major second-line treatment for ovarian cancer.

NICE GUIDELINES ON THE USE OF CHEMOTHERAPY DRUGS IN OVARIAN CANCER

Use of taxanes

NICE has issued guidelines on the use of taxanes in ovarian cancer. These state that the use of paclitaxel in combination with a platinum agent, i.e. cisplatin or carboplatin, should be standard initial therapy in patients after surgery.

The combination of paclitaxel and a platinum agent can be used in recurrent disease if this combination has not already been given. Randomised controlled trials have shown that the combination of paclitaxel with a platinum agent increases median survival by 10 months, with quality of life not significantly differing to platinum treatment alone.

Topotecan (NICE 2001/028)

Topotecan prevents DNA replication by inhibiting the enzyme topoisomerase I. It is recommended in women with advanced ovarian cancer if first-line chemotherapy has not been successful. It is not recommended in women with an ECOG score of 3 or less or in those who have previously received topotecan.

Pegylated liposomal doxorubicin hydrochloride

Pegylated liposomal doxorubicin hydrochloride (PLDH) is recommended as an option for the treatment of women with advanced ovarian cancer. This is to be used after treatment with a platinum agent. The principle of encapsulating doxorubicin in liposomes that have a surface-bound glycol is that the blood circulation time increases before metabolism. There is an increase in the delivery of drug to the target cancer cells and anticipated reduced toxicity. It is given intravenously and toxicities include painful skin rashes, including on the palms and soles of the feet; these patients may also suffer from cardiac toxicity. Patients in whom this drug is not indicated are those with a low performance status or bowel obstruction. Phase II response rates still remain low and are similar to topotecan as second-line treatment with advanced ovarian cancer.

PANCREATIC CANCER

Most patients with pancreatic cancers still die of their disease, despite improvements in surgical techniques, postoperative supportive care and the introduction of adjuvant chemotherapy and radiation. This is often due to the poor responses of these malignancies to current chemotherapeutic regimens. Pancreatic cancer accounts for 4% of cancer deaths, with over three-quarters of patients presenting with metastatic disease.

Cigarette smoking is the most reliably linked risk factor, although diet, caffeine, alcohol, chronic pancreatitis and diabetes have also been associated with the development of pancreatic cancer. Most of these tumours are adenocarcinomas occurring within the head of the pancreas. There is a TNM staging for this cancer but perhaps a simpler way is to describe the status as local or resectable disease, locally advanced unresectable disease or metastatic disease to the liver, peritoneum and lung.

Up to 20% of patients with resectable pancreatic cancer undergo pancreaticoduodenectomy. These are patients without evidence of involvement of surrounding structures such as the superior mesenteric artery and no evidence of distant metastases. The 5-year survival can be up to 20% (Li 2004). There is debate about the value of adjuvant fluorouracil-based chemoradiation against chemotherapy alone, the former being used more in the USA rather than in Europe (Neoptolemos 2001).

Locally advanced disease is defined as when the tumour spreads to surrounding blood vessels or adjacent structures such as the superior mesenteric artery and coeliac axis but with no distant spread. The combination of fluorouracil plus radiotherapy gives a median survival of around 10 months, with a high chance of local relapse The use of 5-FU in combination with radiation in the locally advanced setting has been shown to give response rates of 15–28%; this is the standard care. Studies of combinations of 5-FU and other agents, such as doxorubicin and cisplatin, showed greater toxicity and no significant improvement in survival with little clinical benefit. However, the aim in this group of patients particularly must be to palliate symptoms, although the majority of these patients develop progressive or metastatic disease within months and are inoperable.

Chemotherapy for advanced and metastatic pancreatic cancer (spread to liver, lungs, etc.) is palliative. These patients will suffer from a range of symptoms, including weight loss, pain and anorexia, together with intractable ascites. Gemcitabine has emerged as the cornerstone of current chemotherapy for pancreatic cancer based on the results of a randomised trial comparing it with 5-FU in patients with advanced unresectable disease. Median survival still remains low, at around 5 months. Randomised trials looking at quality of life issues such as pain, functional impairment and weight loss have shown statistically significant response rates of over 20% of patients with gemcitabine compared with responses of 5% with 5-FU alone (Heinemann 2002). Survival and objective response were secondary endpoints. Gemcitabine has also shown activity in pancreatic cancer refractory to 5-FU and seems to produce a similar clinical benefit response when it is used as first-line therapy.

Combination therapies of gemcitabine and cisplatin, or irinotecan, or oxaliplatin compared to gemcitabine alone have shown variable response rates sometimes better than gemcitabine alone, but with no real appreciable increase in median survival time.

In summary, gemcitabine is the standard of care in metastatic pancreatic cancer, offering a slightly better overall survival than 5-FU. Current gemcitabine- or 5-FU-containing combinations may result in longer survival times than those seen with single-agent therapy; however, results to date remain preliminary.

PROSTATE CANCER

The incidence of prostate cancer is rising and it is the second most common malignancy in men in the UK and USA. There is a genetic component and around 5% of cases are hereditary. Loss of the tumour suppressor gene p53 is one of the molecular changes that have been documented. The predominant histological type is adenocarcinoma. The normal architecture is lost in malignancy and the Gleason pathological grading system takes into account and scores the two most common forms of glandular histology. It correlates with prognosis in localised prostatic cancer (Agarwal & Waxman 2002) in that Gleason scores of 7–10 have a 10% greater chance per year of developing metastases compared to a score of 2–4. In prostate cancer there is release of the tumour marker prostate-specific antigen (PSA) from the cell cytoplasm.

This can be used to determine response to treatment both from androgen deprivation as well as from the use of chemotherapy. Transrectal ultrasound-guided biopsy of the prostate is used to aid diagnosis and the majority are adenocarcinoma.

The natural history of prostate cancer is variable but factors thought to be of prognostic importance include the PSA at the time of diagnosis, the Gleason score and the TNM stage (Table 5.16) (Agarwal & Waxman 2002). In some cases it is difficult to decide whether to treat because patients might be completely asymptomatic with localised disease with a long natural history of the disease.

STAGE I AND II DISEASE

These are patients with organ-confined disease. There is controversy over when and how to treat this disease because patients might be completely unaware of its presence. Modalities of treatment that have been considered include radical prostatectomy, radiotherapy, hormone therapy or surveillance alone. Younger patients do tend to get local therapy because a significant proportion (< 20%) may develop progressive disease. Radical prostatectomy or radiotherapy is generally offered to patients with stage II disease, although there have not been many randomised trials comparing the differences in terms of outcome between the two modalities of treatment. A rising PSA after treatment warrants further investigation to exclude recurrent or progressive disease.

As most patients may be asymptomatic, the choice of treatment is important because side effects of treatment should be considered, such as proctitis and loss of potency after radiotherapy. The use of hormonal therapy in stages I and II disease is usually through clinical trial use.

STAGES III AND IV LOCALLY ADVANCED PROSTATE CANCER

Tumours such as T3 or T4, N0, N1 or N2 and M0 invade local structures and involve regional lymph nodes. Survival rates may be 30% at 15 years. Radiotherapy is the mainstay of treatment, together with adjuvant hormone ablation (e.g. using LHRH analogues); however, there still remains some controversy about the best modality of treatment.

STAGE IV ADVANCED, METASTATIC DISEASE

The standard treatment for metastatic disease is hormone ablation. The drug that was used for many years was diethylstilboestrol but this has been superseded by new, more effective drugs. The use of LHRH agonists in this setting has been well documented in randomised controlled trials, although

TABLE 5.16 Staging of prostate cancer (AJCC 1997) (Reproduced with kind permission)

Grade	Description
Tumour (T)	
T0	No tumour
T1	No clinical evidence through palpation or imaging
T1a	Incidental tumour in ≤ 5% of resected tissue
T1b	Incidental tumour in > 5% of resected tissue
T1c	Raised PSA led to finding tumour by transrectal biopsy
T2	
T2a	Tumour confined to one lobe only
T2b	Tumour involves both lobes
T3	
T3a	Unilateral or bilateral extra capsular extension
T3b	Tumour invades seminal vesicles
T4	Tumour fixed or invades bladder neck, external sphincter, rectum, levator muscles and /or pelvis
Lymph node (N)	
N0	No regional nodes
N1	Regional node metastases
Metastases (M)	
M0	No distant metastases
M1a	Non-regional node metastases
M1b	Bone metastases
M1c	Other metastases
Stage	
Stage I	T1a, N0, M0, Gleason score 2–4
Stage II	T1a, N0, M0, Gleason score ≥ 5 T1b, T1c, T2, N0, M0
Stage III	T3, N0, M0
Stage IV	T4, N0, M0 T4, N0, M0 Any T, N1, M0 Any T, any N, M1

the aim of treatment is for palliation rather than curative intent. The use of antiandrogen therapy, such as cyproterone acetate, is mandatory – usually for 3 weeks before the use of LHRH analogues to prevent 'tumour flare', which represents an initial surge of LH. The aim of LHRH treatment is to reduce testosterone production to the equivalent of a medical castration and this takes around a month to achieve. The drug is administered subcutaneously and 1-month and 3-month depot formulations are available.

Side effects include loss of libido, hot flushes and the risk of osteoporosis. Other options are to use the antiandrogens flutamide or bicalutamide. The latter is a once-daily, long-acting oral dose, which is of value in non-metastatic disease but probably no more effective than medical or surgical castration in metastatic disease. Side effects include gynaecomastia, although the majority of patients have preservation of potency. The combination of both an antiandrogen and the use of medical castration (i.e. LHRH agonist) or surgical castration (orchidectomy) have not been shown to be superior to androgen blockade alone in metastatic prostatic cancer. There is evidence that the early use of hormonal therapy in this setting may prolong survival and reduce disease recurrence. The switching to a different antiandrogen is advocated in the presence of disease progression.

Patients have a median time to progression of around 18 months with androgen deprivation. 'Hormone-refractory disease' refers to those patients who have progressed after total androgen deprivation. In the presence of disease progression, withdrawal of antiandrogen therapy leads to a drop in the PSA in up to 50% of patients; this lasts for around 3 months.

Radiotherapy is particularly useful in patients with bone pain as a means of palliating symptoms. The use of strontium as an alternative for the treatment of bone metastasis has also been encouraging. The use of single-agent chemotherapy has been disappointing, with drugs such as carboplatin, cisplatin, doxorubicin, cyclophosphamide, estramustine and mitoxantrone showing response rates that are less than 20% at best.

In patients who have relapsed and have had antiandrogen therapy withdrawn, with some effect, or if, despite withdrawal, there is evidence of disease progression, then the combination of corticosteroids and mitoxantrone chemotherapy has been shown to give a response rate of up to 30% with an improvement in pain control and quality of life scores. This compares with 12% for corticosteroids alone. Toxicity of treatment is mild with grade I myelosuppression, emesis, alopecia and cardiomyopathy.

The recent trials of Taxotere® have been particularly encouraging, with response rates between 20 and 30%. Recent trials comparing Taxotere® and steroids against mitoxantrone and steroids show that Taxotere® had a survival benefit of 3 months, with improved quality of life in patients with metastatic-hormone-refractory patients (Tannock et al 2004). The median survival was 16.5 months in the mitoxantrone group compared to

Prostate cancer: case 1

A 69-year-old man with symptoms of prostatism was referred up after a finding of a raised PSA of 35 ng/mL. He underwent transrectal ultrasound prostatic biopsy and his biopsies showed poorly differentiated Gleason 5 + 5 tumour in all his prostatic sections. In view of his elevated PSA and symptoms it was felt that he would benefit from hormonal suppression. Treatment was prescribed with 2 weeks of cyproterone at a dose of 200 mg tds followed by luteinising hormone-releasing hormone antagonist therapy and Zoladex® 3-monthly subcutaneous injection at a dose of 10.8 mg. There was good reduction in the PSA to 3 ng/mL after 6 months' treatment.

Comment

The Gleason score defines the histological grading of prostate cancer and is used to assess the prognosis of the disease. The Gleason grading system defines cell size and shape and the level of cell differentiation. Grade 1 defines less aggressive disease whereas grade 5 is the most aggressive. As biopsies can show heterogeneity in terms of the cell grading, the two most prominent grades are added to give the Gleason score. Scores above 4 are prognostically worse, with greater likelihood of metastatic spread. The most common pathology is adenocarcinoma of the prostate:

- grade 1: small round glands, well-defined edges
- grade 2: simple round glands, loosely packed, loosely defined edges
- grade 3: variation in glandular size and organisation with ill-defined infiltrating edges
- grade 4: atypical cells with extensive infiltration of stromal and neighbouring tissues
- grade 5: undifferentiated sheets of cancer cells.

Cyproterone is given before LHRH therapy in prostate cancer to stop so-called 'tumour flare'. LHRH treatment can initially lead to a rise in testosterone levels, which in turn can lead to an increase in the size of tumours. Spinal cord compression following treatment has been reported. Cyproterone is used as an antiandrogen to lower testosterone levels. Other side effects include hot flushes, loss of libido, impotence, breast tenderness, skin rashes and musculoskeletal pain (which can be treated with NSAIDs).

18.9 months in the group given Taxotere® every 3 weeks. There was no significant survival benefit in giving weekly Taxotere®. Just under 50% of men in the Taxotere® group had at least a 50% decrease in the serum PSA level, with reductions in pain and improvements in the quality of life. There was some degree of toxicity associated with the Taxotere® group.

RENAL CELL TUMOURS

This cancer originates from the proximal tubular cells and accounts for 3000 deaths in the UK and has increased in incidence by 20% in the last 10 years. Associations include cigarette smoking and obesity.

Patients with this cancer often present with non-specific symptoms: back pain, weight loss, fatigue, anaemia and haematuria being the most common. These are the most common presenting symptoms of kidney cancer. There are some familial conditions, including von Hippel–Landau disease, which is an autosomal dominant condition associated with multiple tumours.

Prognosis depends on how localised the disease is, how big the tumour is, the histology and the cytogenetics of the disease. The overall survival rate is around 50% at 10 years. Stage I and II tumours have localised disease to the fascia around the kidneys, whereas stages III and IV involve invasion to surrounding organs such as the renal vein, vena cava, lymph nodes and distant organs such as bone, distant nodes, liver and lung. Stage II cancers can have a 5-year survival of over 60%, whereas stage IV cancers may have a survival rate of less than 1 year.

TREATMENT

The treatment for localised stage I and II tumours is radical nephrectomy. Partial nephrectomy is considered in selective cases and local relapses may require further surgery, although patients may present with metastatic disease. The use of adjuvant therapy is not standard practice and clinical trials are ongoing to best define its role.

Some patients with stage III disease may benefit from nephrectomy, although a significant proportion present with frankly invasive disease. Similarly, some stage IV patients may undergo nephrectomy or excision of tumour to reduce tumour bulk although the majority of these patients are treated with systemic therapy. The role of standard chemotherapy is minimal, with low responses because of the presence of drug resistance genes in the cancer cells (Vogelzang 1998). The use of immunotherapy has reported some success.

The role of immunotherapy

Interferon-α and interleukin-2 treatments have shown interesting response rates particularly in metastatic disease. With interferon-α, the overall response rate is around 10%, with a complete response in 1% of cases. Interleukin-2 treatment has given response rates of 15–30% in advanced disease.

Interferon-α has a licence in the UK for recurrent or metastatic renal cell carcinoma, whereas recombinant interleukin-2 is licensed for metastatic renal cell carcinoma.

Randomised trials have shown a survival advantage with interferon-α in patients with metastatic disease. Median survival averages 11.6 months and

2-year survival averages 22% (Coppin 2000). It is usually given as a subcutaneous injection three times a week and toxicities of treatment include flu-like symptoms, cardiovascular toxicity such as arrhythmias and hypotension, as well as low-grade myelosuppression, hepatotoxicity and mood changes leading to depression.

Interleukin-2 has a similar response rate to interferon-α but no survival advantage (Atkins 2004). It is also given as a subcutaneous injection but is contraindicated if a patient has a performance status higher than 1, more than one organ affected by metastases and less than 2 years from diagnosis to consideration of treatment. Toxicities include myelosuppression and central nervous system toxicity.

The combination of interleukin-2 and interferon-α has not been shown to give a higher survival benefit.

The future management of this cancer may be based on novel therapies such as dendritic-cell-derived vaccines. Dendritic cells are white blood cells that activate T cells through antigen presentation. Vaccines based on cultured dendritic cells into which RNA from a renal cancer patient's own tumour is introduced have been developed. The dendritic cells use the RNA for antigen presentation to activate T cells. Early clinical studies to date have shown that vaccination was well tolerated without significant toxicity. There has been early evidence of immunological responses and some evidence of disease response in patients with advanced disease (Avigan 2004). Other approaches such as monoclonal antibodies and gene therapy and allogeneic cell transplantation are being considered.

SOFT TISSUE SARCOMAS

Soft tissue sarcomas are a mixed group of malignant tumours that arise from the mesenchymal tissues; they are rare but the incidence is rising. They demonstrate genetic changes and alteration in gene expression such as mutation of the p53 gene. They usually present with painless lump, usually on the lower extremity although other sites such as the upper extremity can be involved. Radiological investigations by MRI and CT scan are the best modalities to help evaluate stage; histological grading is essential to determine management.

The American Joint Committee on Cancer (AJCC) has devised a staging system for soft tissue sarcomas (Table 5.17).

The mainstay of treatment is surgery and radiotherapy. Grade 1 tumours should be treated with wide or radical surgery alone, which usually allows for good functional outcome. Preoperative or postoperative radiotherapy, depending on the likely surgical outcome, has been used with good results, allowing less radical surgery for selected patients.

Tumours larger than G2–G3 are likely to metastasise. There is controversy about the role of adjuvant chemotherapy. A recent meta-analysis has shown

TABLE 5.17 AJCC staging system for soft tissue sarcoma

Grade	Description
Histology grade	
GX	Grade cannot be assessed
G1	Well differentiated
G2	Moderately differentiated
G3	Poorly differentiated
G4	Undifferentiated
Tumour (T)	
T	Primary tumour
Tx	Primary tumour cannot be assessed
T0	No evidence of primary tumour
T1	Tumour 5 cm or less in greatest dimension
T1a	Superficial tumour
T1b	Deep tumour
T2	Tumour greater than 5 cm in greatest dimension
T2a	Superficial tumour
T2b	Deep tumour
Lymph node (N)	
N	Regional lymph nodes
Nx	Regional lymph nodes cannot be assessed
N0	No histological verified metastases to regional lymph nodes
N1	Histologically verified regional lymph-node metastases
Metastases (M)	
M	Distant metastases
Mx	Distant metastases cannot be assessed
M0	No distant metastases
M1	Distant metastases
Stage I	
A	Low-grade, small superficial and deep: G1–2, T1a–1b, N0, M0
B	Low-grade, large, superficial: G1–2, T2a, N0, M0

continued on page 146

TABLE 5.17 AJCC staging system for soft tissue sarcoma *continued*

Grade	Description
Stage II	
A	Low-grade, large, deep: G1–2, T2b, N0, M0
B	High-grade, small, superficial and deep: G3–4, T1a–1b, N0, M0
C	High-grade, large, superficial
Stage III	High-grade, large, deep: G3–4, T2b, N0, M0
Stage IV	Any metastasis: any G, any T, N1, M0; any G, any T, N0, M1

that doxorubicin-based chemotherapy leads to a gain in the recurrence-free survival from 45–55%, with a small gain in overall survival. In adults with localised resectable soft tissue sarcoma, doxorubicin-based adjuvant chemotherapy leads to a significantly improved time to local and distant recurrence and overall recurrence-free survival with a degree of improved overall survival (Sarcoma Meta-analysis Collaboration 2000). To better define the role of adjuvant therapy the Soft Tissue and Bone Sarcoma Group (STBSG) of the EORTC is to coordinate a randomised trial of adjuvant chemotherapy in high-grade primary or recurrent soft tissue sarcoma at any site with surgery used as primary therapy (Issels 2002).

The two most active agents in metastatic disease are ifosfamide and doxorubicin. In adults with locally advanced or metastatic soft tissue sarcoma who require palliative chemotherapy, single-agent doxorubicin is better tolerated than combination chemotherapy in terms of toxicity and there is no difference in terms of survival outcome data (Bramwell 2003). Response rates for doxorubicin have been around 25% in this group of patients. The median survival for patients with metastatic disease is usually around 12 months. Single-agent doxorubicin has moderate myelosuppression, alopecia and emesis as its side effect profile and the risk of cardiomyopathy increases with cumulative use. Ifosfamide has a similar response rate and toxicity profile, which also includes haemorrhagic cystitis and nephrotoxicity. The combination of ifosfamide and doxorubicin gives a wider toxicity profile with not much more gain in terms of response rates than single-agent doxorubicin.

KAPOSI'S SARCOMA

AIDS is an example of an immune deficiency state in which there is an increased risk of cancer. Kaposi's sarcoma together with high-grade, B-cell non-Hodgkin's lymphoma is the predominant AIDS-defining malignant disease. Classic Kaposi's sarcoma usually starts as a flat, blue–red lesion that can progress to plaque formation; it is usually treated with radiotherapy or surgery. A small proportion of renal transplanted patients may also develop this disease and is associated with immunosuppression. Chemotherapy with single agents such as paclitaxel or immunotherapy are used for advanced disease.

TESTICULAR CANCER

In the UK, testicular germ tumours account for less than 1500 new cases and account for 1% of all cancers in men. Interplay between genetics and environmental factors triggers the development of these tumours at an early age. Presentation may be typical (painless testicular lumps, aching in the scrotal area) or atypical, with symptoms of metastatic disease, e.g. haemoptysis. Delays in diagnosis adversely affect prognosis but 80% of men with metastatic testicular cancer are cured. This, however, depends on early presentation and men who present within 1 month of noticing a testicular lump are curable with a radical inguinal orchidectomy alone.

Tumour markers that help diagnosis and follow-up include α-fetoprotein (AFP), β-hCG and LDH. Metastatic spread is either via the lymphatics to the para-aortic nodes or haematogenous spread to liver, lung and brain (Schmoll 2004). Thus serum tumour markers and chest X-rays initially, together with a CT scan of the chest, abdomen and pelvis particularly, constitute the staging investigations, which also need to be done as follow-up after definitive therapy. Germ cell tumours account for over 95% of malignant testicular cancers.

The Royal Marsden Hospital has devised a staging system for testicular cancer (Dearnley et al 2001) (Table 5.18).

Treatment varies for the histological type of tumour divided into either seminomas or non-seminomatous (teratomas).

TABLE 5.18 Staging for testicular cancer: the Royal Marsden Hospital staging system for testicular cancer (Dearnley et al 2001) (Reproduced with kind permission)

Stage	Description
I	No metastases, either clinically or radiological
II	Abdominal metastasis
III	Supradiaphragmatic nodal metastasis
IV	Lung metastases

STAGE I SEMINOMAS

Orchidectomy and adjuvant para-aortic radiotherapy remain the mainstay of treatment and three-quarters of men with seminomas receive this treatment. They are offered the possibility of storing sperm before treatment commences, and a prosthesis. The cure rate is 95% and this group is followed up with surveillance monitoring with tumour markers, X-ray and CT scans.

STAGE I NON-SEMINOMATOUS

Stage I non-seminomatous tumours with a high risk of vascular invasion receive either adjuvant chemotherapy containing cisplatin or surveillance with monthly chest X-rays and tumour marker measurement after orchidectomy and retroperitoneal node dissection (Cullen 1996). The prognosis remains excellent with a cure rate of 95%.

OPTIONS IN STAGE II–IV DISEASE

Stage II seminomatous

- The cure rate is 85–95%.
- Non-bulky disease: radical inguinal orchidectomy followed by radiation to the retroperitoneal and ipsilateral pelvic lymph nodes.
- Bulky disease (= 5 cm): radical inguinal orchidectomy followed by cisplatin combination chemotherapy or radiation to the abdominal and pelvic lymph nodes. Recurrence rate is higher after radiation for bulky stage II and chemotherapy is considered.

Stage II non-seminomatous

- Can achieve cure rates of 95%.
- Treatment is by radical inguinal orchidectomy, removal of retroperitoneal lymph nodes and combination chemotherapy.

All patients need surveillance and the option of surgical removal of residual tissue after treatment is controversial.

Stage III seminomatous

- Cure rates of 90% achieved.
- Radical inguinal orchidectomy with combination chemotherapy.
- Management of residual tissue remains controversial.

Stage III non-seminomatous

- 70% cured by combination chemotherapy followed by the option of surgical removal of the testis.

In patients with stage II–IV seminomatous metastatic disease, high-volume disease and metastatic non-seminomatous disease, the mainstay of treatment is with chemotherapy consisting of bleomycin, etoposide and cisplatin (BEP). The number of courses varies with prognostic factors (site of spread, tumour markers, testicular size). In a randomised multicentre trial evaluating the efficacy of carboplatin plus etoposide and bleomycin (CEB) versus cisplatin plus etoposide and bleomycin (BEP) in first-line chemotherapy of patients with good-risk non-seminomatous germ cell tumours, the BEP regimen was effective in the treatment of patients. The trial demonstrated that the regimen containing carboplatin was not as efficacious as that containing cisplatin (Horwich et al 1997).

In good-prognosis germ cell cancer it has been shown that three versus four cycles of bleomycin, etoposide and cisplatin (BEP) and the 5-day schedule versus the 3-day schedule per cycle are equivalent. Giving chemotherapy in 3 days again did not lessen the effectiveness of the chemotherapy regimen (de Wit 2001).

The prognosis in early metastatic disease remains good for both groups, with 5-year survival rates varying from 85% for seminomas and over 90% for non-seminomatous disease. The International Germ Cell Consensus Classification (1997) lists clinically based prognostic factors that are relevant for metastatic germ cell tumours. It was advocated for use in clinical trial work to facilitate collaboration between trial centres. The group assessed data from over 5000 patients treated with cisplatin-based chemotherapy for metastatic germ cell tumours, with a median follow-up of over 5 years. Important adverse prognostic factors were as follows:

- Non-seminomatous germ cell tumours:
  - involvement of the mediastinal as the primary site
  - the degree of elevation of AFP, hCG and LDH
  - the presence of non-pulmonary visceral metastases, e.g. liver, bone and brain.
- Seminomas:
  - the involvement of non-pulmonary visceral metastases was the main prognostic factor, along with a normal AFP level.
- Combining the groups:
  - a good prognosis tumour is defined as a 90% 5-year survival
  - a poor prognosis has a close-to 50% 5-year survival rate.

An added factor that must be taken into account is that the centre where treatment takes place must have a good prognostic outlook. There is an association between how experienced the treating institution is with metastatic poor-prognosis non-seminoma disease and the long-term clinical outcome of the patients (Collette 1999). As the majority of cases are curable, the long-term effects of receiving chemotherapy must be monitored. These patients are at risk of nephrotoxicity, ototoxicity, secondary leukaemias and infertility.

In patients who have recurrent disease, treatment is dependent on the cancer type, the treatment received and the site of recurrence. Salvage chemotherapy includes the IPE regimen (ifosfamide, cisplatin and etoposide), which can lead to a 25% complete response rate. Another option is the use of high-dose chemotherapy with autologous marrow transplantation in refractory disease. This may lead to complete remissions in up to 20% of patients. In some selected patients the remission rate may be as high as 50% in good prognostic groups. Some patients may relapse after 2 years of complete remission and in this group some do better with surgical treatment of residual disease.

THYROID CANCER

In the UK there are just under 1000 new cases, with 220 deaths per year, accounting for around 1% of all new malignant disease; 94% of these are well differentiated thyroid cancers consisting of follicular or papillary thyroid cancers. The rest are medullary thyroid cancers (5%), neuroendocrine and anaplastic thyroid cancers (91%).

The British Thyroid Associations advocate the need for better management of these cancers. Up to 10% of patients diagnosed with thyroid cancer die of their disease. There are certain poor prognostic factors, which include greater age, male sex, poorly differentiated tumours and advanced stage of tumour. The drive is that these cancers are treated in regional centres with designated multidisciplinary teams.

The mainstay of treatment for the majority of cases is surgery (e.g. total thyroidectomy) followed by adjuvant radioiodine treatment and thyroid hormone replacement therapy. Disease monitoring uses serum thyroglobulin to diagnose recurrent disease. In metastatic disease, surgical resection and the use of radioactive iodine are advocated. If surgical resection is not possible, say, for locally invasive disease, then external beam radiotherapy is offered. The role of chemotherapy is limited. Doxorubicin is associated with response rates of up to 40% for progressive differentiated cancers unresponsive to radioactive iodine. Combination therapies simply add toxicity without much in the way of response and there is no evidence that survival is improved.

References

Bladder cancer

Advanced Bladder Cancer (ABC) Meta-analysis Collaboration 2003 Neoadjuvant chemotherapy in invasive bladder cancer: a systematic review and meta-analysis. Lancet 361:1927–1934
This meta-analysis looked at over 2000 from ten randomised trials and showed that platinum-based combination chemotherapy confers a significant benefit to overall survival, with a 13% reduction in risk of death and an overall survival increase from 45% to 50%.

Alexandroff AB et al 1999 BCG immunotherapy of bladder cancer: 20 years on. Lancet 353:1689–1694

Herr HW 1998 Neoadjuvant chemotherapy and bladder-sparing surgery for invasive bladder cancer: ten-year outcome. Journal of Clinical Oncology 4:1298–1301

Hussain SA, James ND 2003 The systemic treatment of advanced and metastatic bladder cancer. Lancet Oncology 8:489–497

This review looks at the role of chemotherapy in metastatic disease when median survival is about 1 year. It advocates the role of platinum drugs in studies of combination chemotherapy regimens and looks at the role of taxanes, gemcitabine and ifosfamide as part of combination therapy with the platinum agents. It advocates the use of molecular prognostic markers into phase II and III trials.

International Collaboration of Trialists (on behalf of the Medical Research Council Advanced Bladder Cancer Working Party, EORTC Genito-Urinary Group, Australian Bladder Cancer Study Group, National Cancer Institute of Canada Clinical Trials Group, Finnbladder, Norwegian Bladder Cancer Study Group, and Club Urologico Espanol de Tratamiento Oncologico (CUETO) Group) 2000 Neoadjuvant cisplatin, methotrexate and vinblastine chemotherapy for muscle-invasive bladder cancer: a randomised controlled trial. Lancet 354:533–540

In this study, patients with T2, G3, T3, T4a, N0–Nx or M0 transitional cell carcinoma of the bladder who were undergoing curative cystectomy or full-dose external-beam radiotherapy were randomly assigned three cycles of neoadjuvant chemotherapy (cisplatin, methotrexate, and vinblastine, with folinic acid rescue) or no chemotherapy. The primary aim was to see if a 10% improvement in 3-year survival could be achieved with this chemotherapy regimen. Median survival in the chemotherapy group was 44 months compared with 37.5 months for the no-chemotherapy group. This translates to a 5.5% survival advantage. However, over 30% of cystectomy samples contained no tumour after neoadjuvant chemotherapy.

Breast cancer

Baum M et al 2003 Anastrozole alone or in combination with tamoxifen versus tamoxifen alone for adjuvant treatment of postmenopausal women with early-stage breast cancer: results of the ATAC (arimidex, tamoxifen alone or in combination) trial efficacy and safety update analyses. Cancer 1 98(9):1802–1810

After a median follow-up of 33 months, this trial demonstrated that in adjuvant endocrine therapy for postmenopausal patients with early-stage breast cancer, anastrozole was superior to tamoxifen in terms of disease-free survival, time to recurrence and incidence of contralateral breast cancer.

Bonneterre J et al 2000 Anastrozole versus tamoxifen as first line therapy for advanced breast cancer in 668 postmenopausal women: results of the Tamoxifen or Arimidex Randomised Group Efficacy and Tolerability Study. Journal of Clinical Oncology 18:3748–3757

The new aromatase inhibitors are being used as first-line therapy for oestrogen-positive metastatic breast cancer and have demonstrated a good duration of response.

Coombes RC et al 2004 A randomized trial of exemestane after two to three years of tamoxifen therapy in postmenopausal women with primary breast cancer. The New England Journal of Medicine 350:1081–1092

Postmenopausal women affected by breast cancer are usually continued on tamoxifen after 2–3 years' use. This double-blind randomised trial has shown that in switching to exemestane women had fewer recurrences than women who stayed on 5 years of tamoxifen alone; switching also demonstrated improved disease-free survival.

Crown J et al 2002 Chemotherapy for metastatic breast cancer – report of a European expert panel. Lancet Oncology 3:719–726

A review and summary of the guidelines treatments in the treatment of metastatic breast cancer.

Early Breast Cancer Trialists' Collaborative Group 1992 Systemic treatment of early breast cancer by hormonal, cytotoxic, or immune therapy: 133 randomised trials involving 31,000 recurrences and 24,000 deaths among 75,000 women. Lancet 339:71–85

This meta-analysis looked at over 100 randomised trials of the use of systemic adjuvant therapy in early breast cancer. It investigated the use of cytotoxic chemotherapy, hormonal agents and other types of therapy and confirmed that the use of adjuvant chemotherapy with more than one agent gave a significant increase in absolute survival and recurrence-free survival, particularly in node-positive patients. Six months of treatment with multiple chemotherapy agents was no worse than 1 year of treatment in terms of survival, and the use of multiple agents was better than single-agent chemotherapy. Death rates were also reduced in premenopausal women.

Early Breast Cancer Trialists' Collaborative Group 2001 Tamoxifen for early breast cancer. Cochrane Database System Review 1:CD000486. Update Software, Oxford
This was the third meta-analysis of the use of tamoxifen in the adjuvant setting in women with early breast cancer. The results confirmed the value of using tamoxifen. Use of adjuvant tamoxifen treatment for a number of years improves the 10-year survival of women with oestrogen-receptor-positive tumours and of women whose tumours are of unknown oestrogen receptor status.

Early Breast Cancer Trialists' Collaborative Group 2002 Multi-agent chemotherapy for early breast cancer. Cochrane Database System Review 1:CD000487. Update Software, Oxford
This was an update on the analysis of women enrolled in randomised controlled trials using multiple chemotherapy agents, including the anthracyclines, as adjuvant treatment for early breast cancer. It concludes that using multiple chemotherapy agents produced an absolute improvement in mortality of between 7 and 11% in 10-year survival for women aged under 50 at presentation with early breast cancer, and of 2–3% for those aged 50–69.

Farquhar C et al 2003a High dose chemotherapy and autologous bone marrow or stem cell transplantation versus conventional chemotherapy for women with early poor prognosis breast cancer. Cochrane Database System Review 1:CD003139. Update Software, Oxford

Farquhar C et al 2003b High dose chemotherapy and autologous bone marrow or stem cell transplantation versus conventional chemotherapy for women with metastatic breast cancer. Cochrane Database System Review 1:CD003142. Update Software, Oxford

Fisher B et al 1990 Postoperative chemotherapy and tamoxifen compared with tamoxifen alone in the treatment of positive node breast cancer patients aged 50 years and older with tumour responsivness to tamoxifen: results from the National Surgical Adjuvant Breast and Bowel Project B-16. Journal of Clinical Oncology 8:1005–1018

Fisher B et al 1998 Tamoxifen for prevention of breast cancer: report of the National Surgical Adjuvant Breast and Bowel Project P-1 Study. Journal of the National Cancer Institute 90:1371–1388
This trial by the National Surgical Adjuvant Breast and Bowel Project (NSABP) showed that tamoxifen could significantly reduce the incidence of invasive and non-invasive breast cancer in high-risk women.

Gaskell DJ et al 1992 Indications for primary tamoxifen therapy in elderly women with breast cancer. British Journal of Cancer 79:1317–1320
In elderly women, tamoxifen has been shown to be as effective in terms of overall survival as mastectomy.

Giordano SH et al 2002 Breast cancer in men. Annals of Internal Medicine 137:678–687

Goss PE et al 2003 A randomized trial of letrozole in postmenopausal women after five years of tamoxifen therapy for early-stage breast cancer. The New England Journal of Medicine 349:1793–1802
This trial showed that, compared with placebo, letrozole therapy after the completion of standard 5 years of tamoxifen treatment significantly improves disease-free survival in postmenopausal women with breast cancer. It was intended that 5 years of letrozole treatment be given but the trial was stopped early – at just after 2 years follow-up – in view of the positive results.

Howell A et al 2004 Comparison of fulvestrant versus tamoxifen for the treatment of advanced breast cancer in postmenopausal women previously untreated with endocrine therapy: a multinational, double-blind, randomized trial. Journal of Clinical Oncology 22(9):1605–1613

Fulvestrant is a new oestrogen receptor (ER) antagonist that down-regulates oestrogen receptors and has no agonist effects. This trial compared its effects with tamoxifen in the treatment of advanced breast cancer in postmenopausal women. This was a multicentre, double-blind randomised trial in patients with metastatic/locally advanced breast cancer previously untreated for advanced disease. The results indicated that fulvestrant had similar efficacy to tamoxifen and was well tolerated.

Holmberg L, Anderson H, HABITS Steering and Data-monitoring Committees 2004 HABITS (hormonal replacement therapy after breast cancer – is it safe?) a randomised comparison: trial stopped. Lancet 363(9407):453–455

This randomised clinical trial looked at the use of HRT in women with breast cancer. It was terminated early when it was found that women allocated to the HRT arm had a greater new event of breast cancer. The study showed the relationship between the long-term use of tamoxifen and the development of complications such as cardiac and thromboembolic disease.

Ingle JN et al 1986 Randomised trial of bilateral oophorectomy versus tamoxifen in premenopausal women with metastatic breast cancer. Journal of Clinical Oncology 4:178–185

In premenopausal women, tamoxifen has been shown to be as effective in terms of duration of response as oophorectomy, which was the treatment of choice.

Loprinzi CL et al 2000 Venlafaxine in the management of hot flushes in survivors of breast cancer: a randomised trial. Lancet 356(9247):2025–2026

This was a double-blind, placebo-controlled, randomised trial to assess the efficacy of venlafaxine in women with history of breast cancer in controlling hot flushes. The dose ranged from 75 to 150 mg and the side effects included gastrointestinal side effects. However, there was a reduction in the number of daily hot flushes.

Mouridsen H et al 2001 Superior efficacy of letrozole (Femara®) versus tamoxifen as first-line therapy for postmenopausal women with advanced breast cancer: results of a phase III study of the International Letrozole Breast Cancer Group. Journal of Clinical Oncology 19:2596–2606

Perkins GH, Middleton LP 2003 Breast cancer in men. British Medical Journal 327:239–240

Press MF et al 1997 Her2/neu gene amplification characterised by fluorescence in situ hybridisation: poor prognosis in node-negative breast carcinomas. Journal of Clinical Oncology 15:2894–2904

This study showed that in patients with stage I and II breast cancers those with higher levels of HER2/neu protein had shorter disease-free intervals and overall survival than patients with lower levels.

Rutqvist LE, Mattsson A 1993 The Stockholm Breast Cancer Study Group. Cardiac and thromboembolic morbidity among postmenopausal women with early-stage breast cancer in a randomised trial of adjuvant tamoxifen. Journal of the National Cancer Institute 85:1398–1406

Winer EP et al 2005 American Society of Clinical Oncology Technology Assessment on the use of aromatase inhibitors as adjuvant therapy for postmenopausal women with hormone receptor-positive breast cancer: status report 2004. Journal of Clinical Oncology 23(3):619–629

Recommendations on the use of adjuvant aromatase inhibitors have been made in the USA. Adjuvant therapy with an aromatase inhibitor for postmenopausal women with hormone-receptor-positive breast cancer is recommended, particularly for women who have contraindications to the use of tamoxifen. For all other postmenopausal women, the options are 5 years of aromatase inhibitor treatment or sequential therapy consisting of tamoxifen (for either 2–3 years or 5 years) followed by aromatase inhibitors for 2–3 to 5 years. Aromatase inhibitors are contraindicated in premenopausal women amd women with hormone-receptor-negative tumours.

Cervical cancer

Thomas GM 1999 Improved treatment for cervical cancer: concurrent chemotherapy and radiotherapy. New England Journal of Medicine 340:1198–1200

This editorial describes the results of three trials that demonstrated the advantage of using chemotherapy in combination with radiotherapy for locally advanced cervical cancer.

Williams C 1999 Chemotherapy and radiotherapy for locally advanced cervical cancer. British Medical Journal 318:1161–1162
This editorial refers to the New England Journal of Medicine *paper above. The three trials reported showed a highly significant reduction in the rate of cancer progression and longer disease-free survival for patients receiving cisplatin-based chemotherapy concurrent with radiotherapy. This covered different stages of disease (stages IA–IVA) with different chemotherapy regimens, including cisplatin alone, and different control arms, including radiotherapy.*

Colorectal cancer

Benson AB et al 2004 American Society of Clinical Oncology recommendations on adjuvant chemotherapy for stage II colon cancer. Journal of Clinical Oncology 22(16):3408–3419
In the adjuvant setting it has been shown that the combination of 5-FU and folinic acid increases survival rate after resection of colonic cancer in Dukes' C cancers. The treatment for Dukes' B stage II cancers has been more controversial. The American Society of Clinical Oncology reviewed the literature and found that a literature-based meta-analysis found no evidence of a statistically significant survival benefit of adjuvant chemotherapy for stage II patients. It recommended that some patients with stage II disease could be considered for adjuvant therapy, including those who might have had inadequately sampled nodes, T4 lesions, perforation, or poorly differentiated histology.

Dearnley DP et al 2002 Handbook of adult cancer chemotherapy schedules, 2nd edn. The Royal Marsden NHS Trust, Surrey
The UK Department of Health Cancer Guidance subgroup has confirmed the use of 5-FU and folinic acid for 6 months, typically using an i.v. bolus of leucovorin and 5-FU as a 5-day course every 4 weeks for 5 months for patients with Dukes' C colon cancer.

Madoff RD 2004 Chemoradiotherapy for rectal cancer – when, why, and how? New England Journal of Medicine 351(17):1790–1792

Mead GM 2002 Management of oral mucositis associated with cancer chemotherapy. Lancet 359:815–816

Rich TA 2004 Four decades of continuing innovation with fluorouracil: current and future approaches to fluorouracil chemoradiation therapy. Journal of Clinical Oncology 22(11):2214–2232

Scheithauer W et al 2003 Oral capecitabine as an alternative to i.v. 5-fluorouracil-based adjuvant therapy for colon cancer: safety results of a randomised, phase III trial. Annals of Oncology 12:1735–1743

Endometrial cancer

Braithwaite RS et al 2003 Meta-analysis of vascular and neoplastic events associated with tamoxifen. Journal of General Internal Medicine 18(11):937–947

Jones B 2002 Uterus: treatment of cancer. In: Price P, Sikora K (eds) Treatment of cancer, 4th edn. Arnold, London

Keys HM et al 2004 A phase III trial of surgery with or without adjunctive external pelvic radiation therapy in intermediate risk endometrial adenocarcinoma: a Gynecologic Oncology Group study. Gynecologic Oncology 92(3):744–751. Erratum in: Gynecologic Oncology 2004 94(1):241–242

Rochelle E et al 2004 Risk of malignant mixed Mullerian tumours after tamoxifen therapy for breast cancer. Journal of the National Cancer Institute 96(1):70–74

Gastric cancer

Diaz-Rubio E 2004 New chemotherapeutic advances in pancreatic, colorectal, and gastric cancers. The Oncologist 9(3):282–294

Hermans J et al 1993 Adjuvant therapy after curative resection for gastric cancer: meta-analysis of randomized trials. Journal of Clinical Oncology 11:1441–1447

This meta-analysis looked at randomised controlled trials of the adjuvant use of chemotherapy for gastric cancers comparing postoperative chemotherapy to a control arm. There appeared to be no survival advantage for chemotherapy after, against surgery alone.

Webb A et al 1997 Randomized trial comparing epirubicin, cisplatin, and fluorouracil versus fluorouracil, doxorubicin, and methotrexate in advanced esophagogastric cancer. Journal of Clinical Oncology 15:261–267

This reported on the results of a prospectively randomised study that compared the combination of epirubicin, cisplatin and protracted venous infusion fluorouracil (5-FU) (ECF regimen) with the standard combination of 5-FU, doxorubicin and methotrexate (FAMTX) in previously untreated patients with advanced oesophagogastric cancer. It established that ECF should be considered standard treatment for advanced oesophagogastric cancer. The conclusion was that the ECF regimen resulted in a survival and response advantage and was better tolerated compared with FAMTX chemotherapy.

Gestational trophoblastic disease

Bloss JD, Thigpen JT 2001 In: Perry MC (ed) The chemotherapy source book. Lippincott, Williams, Wilkins, Philadelphia

Newlands ES et al 1999a Results with the EMA/CO (etoposide, methotrexate, actinomycin D, cyclophosphamide, vincristine) regimen in high-risk gestational trophoblastic tumours, 1979 to 1989. British Journal of Obstetrics and Gynaecology 98(6):550–557

Newlands ES et al 1999b Recent advances in gestational trophoblastic disease. Hematology and Oncology Clinics of North America 13(1):225–244

Gliomas

Fine HA et al 1993 Meta-analysis of radiation therapy with and without adjuvant chemotherapy for malignant gliomas in adults. Cancer 71(8):2585–2597

Glioma Meta-analysis Trialists Group 2002 Chemotherapy in adult high-grade glioma: a systematic review and meta-analysis of individual patients' data from 12 randomised trials. Lancet 359:1011–1017

Rampling R 2002 Central nervous system. In: Price P, Sikora K (eds) Treatment of cancer, 4th edn. Arnold, London

van den Bent MJ et al 2003 Phase II study of first-line chemotherapy with temozolomide in recurrent oligodendroglial tumors: the European Organization for Research and Treatment of Cancer Brain Tumor Group Study 26971. Journal of Clinical Oncology 21(13):2525–2528

Head and neck cancers

El-Sayed S, Nelson N 1996 Adjuvant and adjunctive chemotherapy in the management of squamous cell carcinoma of the head and neck region. A meta-analysis of prospective and randomized trials. Journal of Clinical Oncology 14(3):838–847

This meta-analysis looked at the role of adding chemotherapy to local definitive treatment.

Vokes EE et al 1993 Head and neck cancer. New England Journal of Medicine 328(3):184–194

Hepatocellular cancer

Hall AJ, Wild CP 2003 Liver cancer in low and middle income countries. British Medical Journal 326:994–995

Mathurin P 1998 Review article: Overview of medical treatments in unresectable hepatocellular carcinoma—an impossible meta-analysis? Aliment Pharmacol Ther. 2:111–126.

Mathurin P 2003 Meta-analysis: evaluation of adjuvant therapy after curative liver resection for hepatocellular cancer. Alimentary Pharmacology and Therapy 17(10): 1247–1261

A review article giving the results of a meta-analysis.

Hodgkin's disease

British National Lymphoma Investigation, Central Lymphoma Group 2001 ChlVPP alternating with PABlOE is superior to PABlOE alone in the initial treatment of advanced Hodgkin's disease: results of a British National Lymphoma Investigation/Central Lymphoma Group randomized controlled trial. British Journal of Cancer 84(10):1293–1300

Canellos GP et al 1992 Chemotherapy of advanced Hodgkin's disease with MOPP, ABVD, or MOPP alternating with ABVD. New England Journal of Medicine 327:1478–1484

EORTC Lymphoma Cooperative Group and GELA 1999 Trial H9 protocol: prospective controlled trial in clinical stages I–II supradiaphragmatic Hodgkin's disease – evaluation of treatment efficacy (long term) toxicity and quality of life in two different prognostic subgroups. EORTC Lymphoma Cooperative group and GELA, EORTC protocol 20982, Brussels

Lister TA et al 1989 Report of a committee convened to discuss the evaluation and staging of patients with Hodgkin's disease: Cotswolds meeting. Journal of Clinical Oncology 7:1630–1636
This led to a modification of the Ann Arbor classification system.

Loeffler M et al 1998 Meta-analysis of chemotherapy versus combined modality treatment trials in Hodgkin's disease. Journal of Clinical Oncology 16:818–829

Specht L 1998 Influence of more extensive radiotherapy and adjuvant chemotherapy on long-term outcome of early-stage Hodgkin's disease: a meta-analysis of 23 randomized trials involving 3,888 patients. Journal of Clinical Oncology 16:830–843
This meta-analysis showed that using more radiotherapy fields or adding more courses of chemotherapy to radiotherapy in the initial treatment of early-stage Hodgkin's disease aided disease control but had only a small effect on overall survival.

Lung cancer

Carney DN 2002 Lung cancer – time to move on from chemotherapy. New England Journal of Medicine 346:126–128

Dearnley DP et al 2002 Handbook of adult cancer chemotherapy schedules. The Royal Marsden NHS Trust, Surrey

Non-small-cell Lung Cancer Collaborative Group 1995 Chemotherapy in non-small cell lung cancer: a metanalysis using updated data on individual patients from 52 randomised trials. British Medical Journal 311:899–909

O'Brien ME 2004 Vinorelbine alternating oral and intravenous plus carboplatin in advanced non-small-cell lung cancer: results of a multicentre phase II study. Annals of Oncology 15(6):921–927

PotterVA et al 2002 In: Price P, Sikora K (eds) Treatment of cancer, 4th edn. Arnold, London

Socinski MA 2004 Cytotoxic chemotherapy in advanced non-small cell lung cancer: a review of standard treatment paradigms. Clinical Cancer Research 10(12 Pt 2): 4210s–4214s

Melanoma and non-melanoma

Balch CM 2001 Final version of the American Joint Committee on Cancer staging system for cutaneous melanoma. Journal of Clinical Oncology 19(16):3635–3648

Lee SM et al 1995 Melanoma: chemotherapy. British Medical Bulletin 51(3): 609–630

Spicer JF, Gore M 2002 Malignant melanoma. In: Price P, Sikora K (eds) Treatment of cancer, 4th edn. Arnold, London

Multiple myeloma

Kyle RA, Arkoma SV 2004 Multiple myeloma. New England Journal of Medicine 351:1860–1873

Myeloma Trialists' Collaborative Group 1998 Combination of chemotherapy versus melphalan plus prednisolone as treatment for multiple myeloma: an overview of 6633 patients from 27 randomised trials. Journal of Clinical Oncology 16: 3832–3842
A review article that focuses on current and new treatments for myeloma.
Sirohi B, Powles R 2004 Multiple myeloma. Lancet 363(9412):875–887
An excellent review of the biology and current treatment of multiple myeloma.

Non-Hodgkin's lymphoma
Czuczman MS 2004 Prolonged clinical and molecular remission in patients with low-grade or follicular non-Hodgkin's lymphoma treated with rituximab plus CHOP chemotherapy: 9-year follow-up. Journal of Clinical Oncology 22(23):4711–4716. Erratum in: Journal of Clinical Oncology 2005 Jan 23(1):248

Oesophageal cancer
Fiorica F et al 2004 Preoperative chemoradiotherapy for oesophageal cancer: a systematic review and meta-analysis. Gut 53(7):925–930
This systemic review of patients with resectable oesophageal cancer demonstrated that chemoradiotherapy plus surgery significantly reduces 3-year mortality compared with surgery alone, but at the expense of increased postoperative mortality.
Malthaner RA et al (the Gastrointestinal Cancer Disease Site Group) 2004 Neoadjuvant or adjuvant therapy for resectable esophageal cancer: a systematic review and meta-analysis. BMC Medicine 2(1):35
This systematic review and meta-analysis assessed the use of neoadjuvant or adjuvant therapy on resectable thoracic oesophageal cancer. Outcome measures were survival, adverse effects and quality of life. Randomised controlled trials that looked at the difference between preoperative and postoperative radiotherapy or chemotherapy against surgery alone were considered. The conclusion was that there is no difference in mortality that surgery should be considered standard practice in resectable tumours.
Medical Research Council Oesophageal Cancer Working Party 2002 Surgical resection with or without preoperative chemotherapy in oesophageal cancer: a randomised controlled trial. Lancet 359(9319):1727–1733
This was a pragmatic randomised trial involving over 800 patients. The primary outcome was survival time in previously untreated patients with resectable oesophageal cancer. Randomisation was to either: 2×4-day cycles, 3 weeks apart, of cisplatin 80 mg/m^2 by infusion (4 hours) with fluorouracil 1000 mg/m^2 daily by continuous infusion for 4 days followed by surgical resection or resection alone. The option of being able to give preoperative radiotherapy was available. Overall survival was better in the chemotherapy arm; 2-year survival rates were 43% and 34%, respectively. The improved survival was not at the expense of additional serious toxicity.
Richel DJ, Vervenne WL 2004 Systemic treatment of oesophageal cancer. European Journal of Gastroenterology and Hepatology 3:249–254

Ovarian cancer
Harries M 2004 A phase II feasibility study of carboplatin followed by sequential weekly paclitaxel and gemcitabine as first-line treatment for ovarian cancer. British Journal of Cancer 91(4):627–632
Harries M, Gore M 2002 Chemotherapy for epithelial ovarian cancer. Lancet Oncology 7:529–545

Pancreatic cancer
Diaz-Rubio E 2004 New chemotherapeutic advances in pancreatic, colorectal, and gastric cancers. The Oncologist 9(3):282–294
Heinemann V 2002 Gemcitabine in the treatment of advanced pancreatic cancer: a comparative analysis of randomized trials. Seminars in Oncology 6(Suppl 20):9–16
Li D et al 2004 Pancreatic cancer. Lancet 363:1049–1057

Neoptolemos JP et al 2001 Adjuvant chemoradiotherapy and chemotherapy in resectable pancreatic cancer: a randomised controlled trial. Lancet 358(9293):1576–1585
The European Study Group for Pancreatic Cancer (ESPAC) assessed the roles of chemoradiotherapy and chemotherapy in a randomised study in the adjuvant setting and results favoured the chemotherapy arm alone.

Prostatic cancer

Agarwal R, Waxman J 2002 Prostate cancer. In: Price P, Sikora K (eds) The treatment of cancer, 4th edn. Arnold, London

American Joint Committee on Cancer (AJCC) 1997 Prostate. In: Fleming ID, Cooper JS, Henson DE et al (eds) AJCC cancer staging manual, 5th edn. Lippincott, Williams, Wilkins, Philadelphia

Renal cell tumours

Atkins MB 2004 Update on the role of interleukin 2 and other cytokines in the treatment of patients with stage IV renal carcinoma. Clinical Cancer Research 10(18 Pt 2): 6342S–6346S

Avigan D 2004 Dendritic cell-tumor fusion vaccines for renal cell carcinoma. Clinical Cancer Research 10(18 Pt 2):6347S–6352S

Coppin C 2000 Immunotherapy for advanced renal cell cancer. Cochrane Database System Review 3:CD001425. Update Software, Oxford

Vogelzang NJ 1998 Kidney cancer. Lancet 352:1691–1696

Soft tissue sarcomas

Bramwell VH 2003 Doxorubicin-based chemotherapy for the palliative treatment of adult patients with locally advanced or metastatic soft tissue sarcoma. Cochrane Database System Review 3:CD003293. Update Software, Oxford

Issels RD 2002 Current trials and new aspects in soft tissue sarcoma of adults. Cancer Chemotherapy and Pharmacology 49(Suppl 1):S4–S8

Sarcoma Meta-analysis Collaboration 2000 Adjuvant chemotherapy for localised resectable soft tissue sarcoma in adults. Cochrane Database System Review 4:CD001419. Update Software, Oxford

Testicular cancer

Collette L et al 1999 Impact of the treating institution on survival of patients with 'poor-prognosis' metastatic nonseminoma. European Organization for Research and Treatment of Cancer Genito-Urinary Tract Cancer Collaborative Group and the Medical Research Council Testicular Cancer Working Party. Journal of the National Cancer Institute 91(10):839–846

Cullen MH et al 1996 Short-course adjuvant chemotherapy in high-risk stage I nonseminomatous germ cell tumors of the testis: a Medical Research Council report. Journal of Clinical Oncology 14(4):1106–1113

Dearnley DP et al 2001 Managing testicular cancer. British Medical Journal 322:1583–1588

de Wit R et al 2001 Equivalence of three or four cycles of bleomycin, etoposide, and cisplatin chemotherapy and of a 3- or 5-day schedule in good-prognosis germ cell cancer: a randomized study of the European Organization for Research and Treatment of Cancer Genitourinary Tract Cancer Cooperative Group and the Medical Research Council. Journal of Clinical Oncology 19(6):1629–1640
This study demonstrated that three cycles of BEP were equivalent to four cycles in good-prognosis germ cell cancer and that giving chemotherapy again in 3 days did not lessen the effectiveness of the chemotherapy regimen.

Horwich A et al 1997 Randomized trial of bleomycin, etoposide, and cisplatin compared with bleomycin, etoposide, and carboplatin in good-prognosis metastatic nonseminomatous germ cell cancer: a multi-institutional Medical Research Council/European Organization for Research and Treatment of Cancer Trial. Journal of Clinical Oncology 5:1844–1852

This randomised, multicentre trial demonstrated the efficacy of cisplatin plus etoposide and bleomycin (BEP) in first-line chemotherapy of patients with good-risk non-seminomatous germ-cell tumours. The BEP regimen was effective in the treatment of patients with good-prognosis metastatic nonseminoma and demonstrated that the regimen containing carboplatin was not as efficacious as that to the cisplatin-containing regimen.

International Germ Cell Consensus Classification 1997 A prognostic factor-based staging system for metastatic germ cell cancers. International Germ Cell Cancer Collaborative Group. Journal of Clinical Oncology 15:594–603

The International Germ Cell Consensus Classification. This document lists clinically based prognostic factors that are relevant for metastatic germ-cell tumours. It was advocated for use in clinical trial work to facilitate collaboration between trial centres. The group assessed data on over 5000 patients treated with cisplatin-based chemotherapy for metastatic germ-cell tumours and with a median follow-up of over 5 years.

Schmoll HJ et al 2004 European consensus on diagnosis and treatment of germ cell cancer: a report of the European Germ Cell Cancer Consensus Group (EGCCCG). Annals of Oncology 9:1377–1399

This European-wide consensus guideline document looks at the available evidence and provides guidelines at each stage for gonadal and extragonadal germ-cell tumours.

Further reading

Cervical cancer

Keys HM 1999 Cisplatin, radiation, and adjuvant hysterectomy compared with radiation and adjuvant hysterectomy for bulky stage IB cervical carcinoma. New England Journal of Medicine 340(15):1154–1161

This randomised, controlled trial looked at the efficacy of radiotherapy given with cisplatin versus radiotherapy alone in women with bulky stage IB cervical cancer. The 3-year survival rates were 83% versus 74%, respectively, although more women had moderate to severe toxicity than with chemotherapy alone. The conclusion was that there was a better overall survival with the combination treatment.

Morris M et al 1999 Pelvic radiation with concurrent chemotherapy compared with pelvic and para-aortic radiation for high-risk cervical cancer. New England Journal of Medicine 340(15):1137–1143.

This randomised, controlled trial looked at the role of radiotherapy alone against radiotherapy given concurrently with cisplatin and fluorouracil chemotherapy in women with stage IIB–IVA cervical cancer. The overall survival rate was 73% for the combination therapy compared with 58% for radiotherapy with a significant difference in disease-free survival (67% versus 40%). The conclusion was that the addition of chemotherapy increased survival.

Neoadjuvant Chemotherapy for Cervical Cancer Meta-Analysis (NACCMA) Collaboration 2004 Neoadjuvant chemotherapy for locally advanced cervix cancer. Cochrane Database System Review CD001774. Update Software, Oxford

This meta-analysis assessed the effect of neoadjuvant chemotherapy followed by radical radiotherapy compared to the same radiotherapy alone; and neoadjuvant chemotherapy followed by surgery compared to radical radiotherapy alone.

Omura GA 1997 Randomized trial of cisplatin versus cisplatin plus mitolactol versus cisplatin plus ifosfamide in advanced squamous carcinoma of the cervix: a Gynecologic Oncology Group study. Journal of Clinical Oncology 15(1):165–171

In women with recurrent disease, the combination of cisplatin and ifosfamide seems to be the favoured regimen. The platinum agents do seem to be able to give an increase in response rate in advanced or recurrent squamous cell cancers. A favourable single agent response is defined as 15% or more for a single agent drug. Ifosfamide has demonstrated response rates of up to 50% in Phase II trials without previous chemotherapy. The most studied platinum based combination has been with ifosfamide.

Rose PG 1999 Concurrent cisplatin-based radiotherapy and chemotherapy for locally advanced cervical cancer. New England Journal of Medicine 340(15):1144–1153

This was a randomised trial of radiotherapy in combination with three concurrent chemotherapy regimens: cisplatin alone; cisplatin, fluorouracil, and hydroxyurea; and hydroxyurea alone in patients with locally advanced cervical cancer with stage IIB, III or IVA disease, without involvement of the para-aortic lymph nodes. The regimens of radiotherapy and chemotherapy that contained cisplatin showed improved rates of survival and progression-free survival.

Tierney JF et al 1999 Can the published data tell us about the effectiveness of neoadjuvant chemotherapy for locally advanced cancer of the uterine cervix? European Journal of Cancer 35(3):406–409

Neoadjuvant therapy refers to the use of chemotherapy before surgery or radiotherapy. This systematic review and meta-analysis looked at 21 randomised trials in the treatment of women with locally advanced cervical cancer. However, it was not possible to use all the trial data for analysis and of the data that was studied there was no clear favourable response data to the use of neoadjuvant chemotherapy.

Whitney CW 1999 Randomised comparison of fluorouracil plus cisplatin versus hydroxyurea as an adjunct to radiation therapy in stage IIB–IVA carcinoma of the cervix with negative para-aortic lymph nodes: a Gynecologic Oncology Group and Southwest Oncology Group study. Journal of Clinical Oncology 17(5): 1339–1348

These patients had tumours staged as IIB, III or IVA. The study demonstrated that patients with locally advanced carcinoma of the cervix had better progression-free survival and overall survival with the combination of 5-FU and cisplatin with radiotherapy.

Waggoner SE 2003 Cervical cancer. Lancet 361:2217–2225

Colorectal cancer

Cancer Guidance Subgroup of the Clinical Outcomes Group 1997. Improving outcomes in colorectal cancer. Department of Health, catalogue nos 97CV0119 and 97 CC0120. HMSO, London

Gastric cancer

Allum WH et al (on behalf of the Association of Upper Gastrointestinal Surgeons of Great Britain and Ireland, the British Society of Gastroenterology, and the British Association of Surgical Oncology) 2004 Guidelines for the management of oesophageal and gastric cancer. Gut 50:v1–v23

These guidelines nicely summarise the evidence to date on the chemotherapy management of gastric cancer. The principal points of interest are that:
* *5-FU is the most active chemotherapeutic agent.*
* *A combination of 5-FU with other agents is superior to single-agent treatment.*
* *The combination of epirubicin, cisplatin and continuous infusion of 5-FU (ECF) appears to be one of the most active regimens.*
* *Adjuvant chemotherapy or chemoradiotherapy is currently not standard practice for resected gastric cancer and should be offered only within the setting of a clinical trial.*
* *The use of intraperitoneal chemotherapy remains investigational.*
* *Neoadjuvant chemotherapy remains investigational with no definite evidence of survival benefit and clinical trials are continuing.*

Hohenberger P, Gretschel S 2003 Gastric cancer. Lancet 362:305–315

Waters JS et al 1999 Long-term survival after epirubicin, cisplatin and fluorouracil for gastric cancer: results of a randomised trial. British Journal of Cancer 80(1–2):269–272

This was a prospective randomised study that compared the combination of epirubicin, cisplatin and protracted venous infusion fluorouracil (ECF regimen) with the standard combination of 5-FU, doxorubicin and methotrexate (FAMTX) in previously untreated patients with advanced oesophagogastric cancer in the neoadjuvant setting (Table 5.4). The trial demonstrated that ECF regimen resulted in a response and survival advantage compared with FAMTX chemotherapy and a greater chance of long-term survival following surgical resection of residual disease is increased with ECF.

Head and neck cancer

Ganly I, Kaye SB 2000 Recurrent squamous-cell carcinoma of the head and neck: overview of current therapy and future prospects. Annals of Oncology 11(1):11–16

Hepatocellular cancer

Schwartz JD et al 2002 Neoadjuvant and adjuvant therapy for resectable hepatocellular carcinoma: review of randomised clinical trials. Lancet Oncology 7:593–602

Hodgkin's disease

Yung L, Linch D 2003 Hodgkin's lymphoma. Lancet 361:943–949

Multiple myeloma

Child JA et al for the Medical Research Council Adult Leukaemia Working Party 2003 High-dose chemotherapy with hematopoietic stem-cell rescue for multiple myeloma. New England Journal of Medicine 348:1875–1883

In this multicentre study (MRC Myeloma VII Trial), patients with previously untreated multiple myeloma who were younger than 65 years of age received standard conventional-dose combination chemotherapy or high-dose therapy and an autologous stem-cell transplant (i.e. intensive therapy with chemotherapy, peripheral blood stem harvesting, high-dose melphalan, reinfusion of stem cells, steroids and maintenance therapy with subcutaneous interferon-α-2A). There was a higher rate of overall survival and progression-free survival in the group receiving high-dose therapy and autologous stem-cell transplant than in the standard-therapy group. The median survival increased by almost 1 year in the high-dose group. The study advocated high-dose therapy with autologous stem-cell rescue as an effective first-line treatment for patients with multiple myeloma who are younger than 65 years of age.

Neuroendocrine tumours

Poston G 2004 GP Fact file. Online. Available at: www.pituitary.org.uk/gp-factfile/index.htm

Non-Hodgkin's lymphoma

Harris NL et al 2000 Lymphoma classification – from controversy to consensus: the REAL and WHO Classification of lymphoid neoplasms. Annals of Oncology 11(suppl 1):S3–S10

Oesophageal cancer

Chau I 2004 Multivariate prognostic factor analysis in locally advanced and metastatic oesophago-gastric cancer – pooled analysis from three multicentre, randomized, controlled trials using individual patient data. Journal of Clinical Oncology 22(12):2395–2403

Using data from over 1000 patients enrolled into randomised controlled trials of patients with locally advanced or metastatic oesophagogastric cancer, it was possible to determine prognostic factors that could aid in the recruitment of patients into trials where they might do well. The four prognostic factors were: performance status, liver metastases, peritoneal metastases and alkaline phosphatase. A prognostic index was determined where patients either had good, moderate or poor risk assessment status if they had no risk factor, one or two risk factors or three or four risk factors respectively. One-year survival for good, moderate, and poor risk groups were 48.5%, 25.7%, and 11%, respectively and the survival differences among these groups were highly significant.

Enzinger PD, Mayer RJ 2003 Oesophageal cancer. New England Journal of Medicine 349:2241–2252

A review article on the diagnosis and management of this cancer.

Ovarian cancer

Background trials and reviews

Advanced Ovarian Cancer Trialists' Group 1998 Chemotherapy in advanced ovarian cancer: four systemic meta-analyses of individual patient data from 37 randomised trials. British Journal of Cancer 78:1479–1487

This meta-analysis was based on patient data from all available randomised controlled trials. The results suggest that platinum-based chemotherapy is better than non-platinum therapy, show a trend in favour of platinum combinations over single-agent platinum, and suggest that cisplatin and carboplatin are equally effective. It concluded by stating that there is no good evidence that cisplatin is more or less effective than carboplatin in any particular subgroup of patients.

Berek JS et al 1999 Advanced epithelial ovarian cancer: 1998 consensus statements. Annals of Oncology 10 (Suppl 1):87–92

The main conclusion drawn by the Consensus Committee was that in previously untreated advanced ovarian cancer, cisplatin plus paclitaxel has been shown to be superior to previous standard therapy with cisplatin plus cyclophosphamide. Carboplatin plus paclitaxel was a reasonable alternative because of toxicity.

Hogberg T et al (SBU Group, Swedish Council of Technology Assessment in Health Care) 2001 A systematic overview of chemotherapy effects in ovarian cancer. Acta Oncologica 40(2–3):340–360

This overview of chemotherapy for epithelial ovarian cancer was based on meta-analysis, randomised controlled trials and prospective studies looking at over 30 000 patients. The main conclusions of the review were:

Stage IA or IB non-clear-cell well-differentiated carcinomas or borderline tumours are low risk if radically operated and there is no indication for adjuvant therapy.

High-risk early ovarian cancer, radically operated (clear cell carcinomas or FIGO stage IA or IB moderately or poorly differentiated carcinomas, or stage IC) have a substantial risk for micrometastatic disease. At this time it was felt that the role of adjuvant chemotherapy was unclear and such therapy should, thus, only be used within clinical trials.

In patients with advanced (FIGO stages II–IV) ovarian cancer paclitaxel/cisplatin was considered to be the standard treatment. This choice of standard therapy, however, was dependent on the ICON 3 study. There were preliminary data supporting the substitution of cisplatin with carboplatin.

Intraperitoneal therapy with cisplatin was not easily accepted treatment. Although high response rates were achieved with high-dose chemotherapy with stem-cell support in the salvage situation the response duration was short.

Hunter RW et al 1992 Meta-analysis of surgery in advanced ovarian cancer: is maximum cytoreductive surgery an independent determinant of prognosis? American Journal of Obstetrics and Gynecology 166:504–511

This meta-analysis showed that maximum cytoreductive surgery was associated with a small increase in median survival time. Platinum-containing chemotherapy improved median survival time substantially and increased dose intensity also conferred a useful survival benefit.

ICON Collaborators 1998 ICON2: randomised trial of single agent carboplatin against the three-drug combination of CAP (cyclophosphamide, doxorubicin and cisplatin) in women with ovarian cancer. Lancet 352:1571–1576

The International Collaborative Ovarian Neoplasm Group, ICON2, was a multicentre international randomised controlled trial looking at whether the three-drug combination of CAP (cyclophosphamide, doxorubicin and cisplatin) was more or less effective than optimal-dose single-agent carboplatin for women with advanced ovarian cancer. The survival curves showed no evidence of a difference between CAP and carboplatin. There was no evidence that CAP or carboplatin were more or less effective in different subgroups, e.g. residual disease. CAP was more toxic than carboplatin. More thrombocytopenia occurred with carboplatin.

International Collaborative Ovarian Neoplasm Group 2002 Paclitaxel plus carboplatin versus standard chemotherapy with single-agent carboplatin or cyclophosphamide, doxorubicin, and cisplatin in women with ovarian cancer: the ICON3 randomised trial. Lancet. 360(9332):505–515

The ICON3 trial. Up to this point, paclitaxel combined with platinum had become a widely accepted treatment for the disease. This trial looked at the safety and efficacy of paclitaxel plus carboplatin with a control of either CAP or carboplatin alone, the primary outcome measure being overall survival. Survival curves showed no evidence of a difference in overall survival between paclitaxel plus carboplatin and control. The median overall survival was 36.1 months on paclitaxel plus carboplatin and 35.4 months on control. Kaplan–Meier curves showed no evidence of a difference between the groups. Paclitaxel plus carboplatin caused more alopecia, fever and sensory neuropathy than carboplatin alone, and more sensory neuropathy than CAP. The conclusion was that single-agent carboplatin and CAP were as effective as paclitaxel plus carboplatin as first-line treatment for women requiring chemotherapy for ovarian cancer. The toxicity profile of single-agent carboplatin made this drug a first-line chemotherapy for ovarian cancer.

McGuire WP et al 1996 Cyclophosphamide and cisplatin compared with paclitaxel and cisplatin in patients with stage III and stage IV ovarian cancer. New England Journal of Medicine 334:1–6

This randomised controlled trial looked at drug combinations in women with advanced ovarian cancer (stage III or IV disease) and residual disease after initial surgery. Toxicity such as allergic reactions were reported more frequently in the cisplatin-paclitaxel group. Progression-free survival was significantly longer in the cisplatin-paclitaxel group (median 18 months) than in the cisplatin-cyclophosphamide group (median 13 months). Survival was also significantly longer in the cisplatin-paclitaxel group (median, 38 versus 24 months).

Ovarian cancer

Buda A et al 2004 Randomised controlled trial comparing single agent paclitaxel vs epidoxorubicin plus paclitaxel in patients with advanced ovarian cancer in early progression after platinum-based chemotherapy: an Italian collaborative study from the Mario Negri Institute, Milan, G.O.N.O. (Gruppo Oncologico Nord Ovest) group and I.O.R. (Istituto Oncologico Romagnolo) group. British Journal of Cancer 90(11):2112–2117

Hofheinz RD et al 2004 Pegylated liposomal doxorubicin in combination with mitomycin C, infusional 5-fluorouracil and sodium folinic acid. A phase-I-study in patients with upper gastrointestinal cancer. British Journal of Cancer 90(10):1893–1897

Pancreatic cancer

Abbruzzese JL 2004 Pancreatic cancer. Lancet 364:1049–1057

Prostatic cancer

Tannock IF et al 2004 The TAX 327 Investigators: docetaxel plus prednisone or mitoxantrone plus prednisone for advanced prostate cancer. New England Journal of Medicine 351(15):1502–1512

Kaposi's sarcoma

Goedert JJ 1998 Spectrum of AIDS-associated malignant disorders. Lancet 351(9119):1833–1839

Testicular cancer

Steele JPC, Oliver TDR 2002 Testicular cancer; perils of very late presentation. Lancet 359:1632–1633

Thyroid cancer

British Thyroid Association (BTA). Online. Available at: www.British-thyroid-association.org

Kendall-Taylor P 2002 Managing differentiated thyroid cancer. British Medical Journal 324:988–989

Sherman SI 2003 Thyroid cancer. Lancet 361:501–511

CHAPTER 6

News and future advances

INTRODUCTION

The aim of current and future drug development programmes is to be able to increase the selectivity of anticancer drugs. That is, to have a therapeutic window in which toxicity of treatment is reduced and minimised. The targets of new drugs are likely to be tumour genes, specific tumour metabolic pathways (such as inhibition of signal transduction pathways) or the prevention of tumour invasiveness and spread. Advances in the understanding of molecular oncology have given insight into how cancer cells are controlled and how the normal cell regulatory processes can become unbalanced (Lane 1998). This knowledge, in combination with pharmacogenomics and pharmacokinetics, will help to lead to selective, tailored therapy to reduce toxicity and improve efficacy. The use of molecular pathology to identify specific tumour characteristics and predicted response to chemotherapy will be critical. New ways of imaging in routine practice will be needed to assess response such as the use of positron emission tomography (PET) in combination with CT scan. Whole-body MRI scans have been shown to be effective at the detection of skeletal metastases. Proof of treatment efficacy will be determined through randomised controlled trials with robust primary outcome data.

EXAMPLES OF NEW TREATMENTS

A good example is the development of new antiangiogenesis agents such as bevacizumab (Avastin®; see colorectal cancer and renal cell cancer). The concept of angiogenesis (the growth of new capillaries from pre-existing vessels) is not new and new drugs are being designed to exploit the many steps in angiogenic tumour development. Some of these steps include:

- Cytokine stimulation of endothelial growth (e.g. vascular endothelial growth factor, VEGF).
- The action of matrix metalloproteinases to degrade extracellular matrix proteins.
- The action of integrins, which help in the migration of endothelial cells.

Examples of targeted drug therapy are given below; these represent a new era in the development of novel anticancer drugs that are going through clinical trials:

- Cetuximab (Erbitux®): for patients with epidermal growth factor receptor (EGFR) overexpression in metastatic colorectal cancer.
- Bortezomib (Velcade®): a proteasome inhibitor. Proteasomes are particles that enable the degradation of endogenous cellular proteins. This drug blocks the proteolytic action of the proteasome. It is used in the treatment of myeloma to stop cell proliferation. It has also been shown to inhibit the bcl-2 gene, allowing cell death by apoptosis, and has been shown to inhibit angiogenesis.
- Gefitinib (Iressa®): an epidermal growth factor receptor-tyrosine kinase (EGFR-TK) inhibitor. Tyrosine kinase is an enzyme that works by adding phosphate groups to special tyrosine amino acids in protein chains. These proteins in turn control cellular communication and growth. The hormones that act on tyrosine kinase receptors are growth factors and hormones that promote cell division such as epidermal growth factor.
- Trastuzumab (Herceptin®): an antibody-based targeted therapy for HER2/neu in overexpressing metastatic breast cancer. Epidermal growth factor is the gene product of the HER2/neu (erb B2) oncogene. Trastuzumab is a recombinant, humanised monoclonal antibody directed against HER2/neu human epidermal growth factor.
- Imatinib mesylate (Gleevec®): for patients with gastrointestinal stromal tumours (see below) and bcr/abl-positive chronic myelogenous leukaemia.

TUMOUR-SPECIFIC EXAMPLES OF NEW DEVELOPMENT IN TREATMENT

BLADDER CANCER

The aim of bladder preservation, particularly in muscle invasive disease, is driving some of the more recent trials using neoadjuvant chemotherapy and concurrent chemoradiation. The use of new drug combinations and new molecular targeted therapy are also being used.

BREAST CANCERS

The development of new hormonal agents in the treatment of breast cancer has been a positive development. Fulvestrant is a new type of oestrogen receptor antagonist. Unlike tamoxifen, it has no agonist effects and it blocks the oestrogen receptor. The advantage of fulvestrant is that it has shown high response rates, particularly against anastrozole, in the treatment of postmenopausal women with advanced breast cancers that have progressed after prior antioestrogenic therapy. However, the role of aromatase inhibitors in postmenopausal women will continue to develop. The role of the new agents such as the taxanes in the adjuvant setting will be evaluated. New technology looking at gene expression will lead to identification of treatment based on target genes.

BRAIN TUMOURS

Ongoing clinical trials in the treatment of gliomas are investigating the role of new drugs in the treatment of glioblastoma multiforme. This aggressive tumour is associated with abnormal angiogenesis and novel agents that block angiogenesis will probably go to clinical trials.

CERVICAL CANCERS

The role of new chemotherapy agents in the management of these patients has yet to be defined. Such agents include the taxanes and capecitabine. The role of chemoradiation and the use of human papilloma virus vaccines are currently being assessed.

COLORECTAL CANCER

New drug combinations with established chemotherapy agents could be an effective way to treat advanced colorectal cancer in the future. The use of oxaliplatin and irinotecan with 5-FU has increased response rates and survival. The types of regimens being used include:

- IFL: irinotecan with bolus 5-FU and leucovorin
- FOLFIRIL: irinotecan and infusional 5-FU with leucovorin
- FOLFOX: oxaliplatin and infusional 5-FU with leucovorin.

The use of targeted agents that are being combined with chemotherapy drugs will be the next stage of development. Bevacizumab is a monoclonal antibody that targets VEGF. VEGF-A is an important angiogenesis signalling factor that is commonly expressed in metastatic colorectal cancer. For example, the use of bevacizumab (Avastin®), an angiogenesis inhibitor, in combination with 5-FU and leucovorin, has shown encouraging results in patients with metastatic colorectal cancer. In one randomised Phase II trial, patients receiving the combination had a more than 50% lower risk of progression than those with standard chemotherapy (Kabbinavar et al 2003). A Phase III, multicentre, double-blind, randomised, placebo-controlled trial (Hurwitz 2004) reported significantly increased response rates, median time to progression and overall survival when bevacizumab is added to the IFL regimen in the first-line treatment of colorectal cancer.

Cetuximab in combination with irinotecan has been evaluated. This combination has shown activity, with cetuximab showing activity in irinotecan-refractory disease (Slevin & Payne 2004). Response rates for cetuximab and irinotecan against cetuximab alone have been around 23% and 11%, respectively, from Phase II trials in patients with advanced disease.

In rectal cancer, novel targeted biological agents, including EGFR inhibitors (Amador & Hidalgo 2004) and VEGF inhibitors, have been shown to enhance the antitumour effect of both radiation and chemotherapy and are currently being explored in initial clinical trials (De Paoli 2004).

The use of these new drugs is likely to be brought forward into the adjuvant setting. The Mosaic adjuvant chemotherapy trial was a large Phase III study of patients with Dukes' B (stage II) and Dukes' C (stage III) colon cancer. The trial looked at the addition of oxaliplatin to standard postoperative adjuvant chemotherapy with fluorouracil and folinic acid and showed that adding oxaliplatin resulted in a reduction in relapse rates of 23% (Slevin & Payne 2004). There was also an increase in disease-free survival.

Trials with these new drugs represent an exciting stage in the management of colorectal cancer and it remains to be seen if overall survival through the use of these drugs in the adjuvant setting is improved.

ENDOMETRIAL CANCER

The role of chemoradiation in the adjuvant setting is one of the focuses of current trials. New drug treatment such as the use of EGFRs will be evaluated.

GALL BLADDER CANCER

Drug combinations with gemcitabine show promise in patients with advanced disease but further randomised trials will be necessary to demonstrate this.

GASTRIC CANCERS

Gastrointestinal stromal tumours

Between 80 and 85% of gastrointestinal stromal tumours (GISTs) have a mutated receptor for a growth factor with tyrosine kinase activity (c-kit). This causes a permanent stimulation of the receptor and leads to uncontrolled cell growth. Imatinib, a tyrosine kinase inhibitor, has shown improved survival in patients with advanced disease who would normally not respond to chemotherapy.

New agent combinations such as capecitabine continue to be tested in gastric cancer with new evaluations of the role of adjuvant therapy and chemoradiation.

HEAD AND NECK CANCERS

Most head and neck cancers overexpress tyrosine kinase receptors. Thus drugs that are going through trials at the moment include the EGFR inhibitors. A new monoclonal antiepidermal growth factor receptor trastuzumab is being evaluated. New chemotherapy agents such as gemcitabine and the taxanes are also being evaluated for this cancer. The role of chemotherapy in combination with radiotherapy remains an area of study.

HEPATOCELLULAR CANCER

One method of improving local concentration of cancer drugs at the tumour site may be through intratumoural delivery of anticancer drugs. One such method being delivered is the use of image-guided, minimally invasive radiofrequency ablation with delivery of chemotherapy agents in high concentrations delivered by biodegradable polymer millirods. These millirods would dissolve and release drugs over predetermined time intervals. Further research and investigation into optimising the doses of drugs delivered and the number of millirods required are necessary but animal models have been encouraging in liver cancer.

HODGKIN'S LYMPHOMA

The use of new chemotherapy agents, such as paclitaxel and gemcitabine, offers new options. The use of immunotoxin therapy may offer a new range of therapy. The principal aim is to maintain high cure rates and reduce secondary toxicity.

LUNG CANCERS

Preclinical development of new molecular targeted agents has led to clinical trials of some of these new agents. These trials include the whole range of new chemotherapy agents, as well as biological therapies and cancer vaccines. For example, the epidermal growth factor receptors (e.g. VEGF) have been targeted in advanced lung cancer.

Gefitinib (Iressa®) is an EGFR-TK inhibitor. It is indicated in the management of patients with locally advanced or metastatic non-small-cell lung cancer and has been used second or third line as an oral formulation given once daily. Clinical trials have shown objective tumour responses and improved disease-related symptoms and quality of life. It was well tolerated, although some concern was raised about pulmonary toxicity.

MELANOMA

The Cancer Genome Project has identified mutations in the BRAF gene in malignant melanoma that could be a potential new target for treatment. The BRAF gene codes for proteins that are important in the signalling pathways that control melanocyte proliferation and differentiation. These mutations were found in two-thirds of primary melanomas. This discovery would open up the possibility of developing drugs that would inhibit the mutant forms of the BRAF genes. Although to date peptide and whole-cell vaccines that generate an immune response through interaction with cell surface proteins have not been successful in metastatic disease, there is ongoing work in the development of allogenic and peptide vaccines. The use of sentinel node biopsy and the combination of chemotherapy with immunotherapy will continue through clinical trials.

PROSTATE CANCER

It is well recognised that when patients with prostate cancer who have advanced or recurrent disease do not respond to hormone treatment that prognosis is poor. Historically, the trials that used chemotherapy for prostate cancer were primarily using single-agent therapy. More recently, combination chemotherapy agents given in the adjuvant and neoadjuvant setting in high-risk patients have been studied in randomised controlled trials. The agents under study include estramustine in combination with paclitaxel, vinblastine or etoposide and future studies will look at how to maximise the potential of new chemotherapy agents in treating this clinically difficult group of patients.

The work using Strontium-89, a β-emitting radioactive analogue, has been encouraging in the treatment of hormone-resistant prostate cancer with painful bone metastases. The relationship between quality of life, survival and bone-targeted treatments are likely to continue, such as further studies on the role of bisphosphonates in metastatic bone disease (Zlotta & Schulman 2001).

New molecular therapeutic therapies are likely to target cell adhesion molecules and assess tumour invasiveness. Immunotherapy in the form of dendritic cell vaccines are showing early clinical promise and seem to be well tolerated, with no significant adverse toxicity reported (Anonymous 2003).

MULTIPLE MYELOMA

New therapeutics for multiple myeloma are likely to be based on new molecular targets (Gahrton 2004). The aim of drug treatment against these targets will be to reduce and inhibit cellular proliferation and induce tumour cellular death. Potential targets include:

• nuclear telomerase inhibitors
• mitochondria, cytoplasm and cell surface molecular targets.

Bortezomib, a proteasome inhibitor, has shown single-agent activity against relapsed and refractory multiple myeloma in both Phase I and II trials. Phase II studies have shown response rates of 35% in advanced myeloma with thrombocytopenia, fatigue and peripheral neuropathy being typical side effects. Clinical trials to date show that combinations using standard chemotherapeutics with bortezomib may have higher response rates. This drug has been approved for use in relapsed myeloma by the FDA in the USA and by the EMEA.

Thalidomide, which has an immunomodulating effect and an antiangiogenic effect, has been studied in Phase II studies in the treatment of relapsed or refractory myeloma. In a study of the combination of thalidomide and dexamethasone the response rate was over 70% (Sirohi & Powles 2004); further trials are ongoing.

Advances in allogenic transplantation techniques have led to improved overall survival. For example, high-dose therapy with melphalan, and autologous stem-cell transplantation, have improved survival from 3 to 5 years (Gahrton 2004).

OVARIAN CANCER

Chemotherapy with the monotherapy alkylating agents was standard therapy for the majority of women with advanced epithelial ovarian cancer until the mid-1980s. The use of cisplatin was incorporated during the 1970s, and combinations of cisplatin and an alkylating agent were widely used during the late 1980s. Paclitaxel in combination with either cisplatin or carboplatin was first-line therapy in ovarian cancer during the 1990s. Currently, research is ongoing into how to use these regimens to maximise response and minimise toxicity and assess new treatments coming through (McGuire & Markman 2003).

The use of new-agent chemotherapy regimens, as well as biological therapies, will dominate research into how to improve survival from this cancer. The technique of using RNA as an interfering mechanism to block the expression of the gene is going to be a useful tool (Downward 2004). Using synthetic small interfering RNA oligonucleotides (siRNA), which can enter the cells by viral vectors and then bind to complementary mRNA sequences in the target gene, can result in blockage of the target gene effect. This RNA technique may be used in the future treatment of ovarian cancer.

RENAL CELL CANCER

Renal cell carcinomas are associated with von Hippel–Lindau tumour suppressor gene inactivation, which in turn is associated with overexpression of VEGR, a protein that stimulates angiogenesis. Bevacizumab is an antibody to VEGF. Early trials in metastatic renal cell carcinoma have shown some promise (Rini & Small 2005). Similarly, overexpression of EGFR has been noted in renal cell cancer and gefitinib has been tested in a Phase II trial but has not shown any significant effect. Other options include the use of vaccines to T-cell targets. A Phase III trial of an autologous antitumour vaccine in patients receiving adjuvant therapy after nephrectomy has shown some early promise.

TESTICULAR CANCER

The importance of surveillance following the treatment of early-stage testicular cancer will continue to be a research area, particularly with the new imaging modalities that may be available for this purpose, such as PET scanning. The use of new drugs with current regimens will be explored, as will the benefit of dose intensity in selected patients.

THYROID CANCER

One of the cellular signalling pathways within the thyroid gland is the ERK pathway. This works to transmit cellular signals from the cell membrane to the nucleus. New drug development will focus on the key processes within this pathway. Other drugs, such as matrix metalloproteinases, may be developed.

References

Colorectal cancer

Amador ML, Hidalgo M 2004 Epidermal growth factor receptor as a therapeutic target for the treatment of colorectal cancer. Clinical Colorectal Cancer 4(1):51–62

De Paoli A 2004 Neoadjuvant therapy of rectal cancer: new treatment perspectives. Tumori 90(4):373–378

Hurwitz H 2004 Integrating the anti-VEGF – a humanized monoclonal antibody bevacizumab with chemotherapy in advanced colorectal cancer. Clinical Colorectal Cancer. 4(Suppl 2):S62–S68

Kabbinavar F et al 2003 Phase II, randomized trial comparing bevacizumab plus fluorouracil (FU)/leucovorin (LV) with FU/LV alone in patients with metastatic colorectal cancer. Journal of Clinical Oncology 21:60–65

Slevin M, Payne S 2004 New treatments for colon cancer. British Medical Journal 329:124–126

Hepatocellular cancer

Reidenbach F 2002 Novel drug delivery device may improve liver cancer outcomes. Lancet Oncology 3:450

Prostate cancer
Anonymous 2003 A second chance for prostate-cancer chemotherapy? Lancet Oncology 4:131
Zlotta AR, Schulman CC 2001 Can survival be prolonged for patients with hormone-resistant prostate cancer? Lancet 357(9253):326–327

Multiple myeloma
Gahrton G 2004 New therapeutic targets in multiple myeloma. Lancet 364:1648–1649
Lane D 1998 The promise of molecular oncology. Lancet 351(Suppl II):17–20
Sirohi B, Powles R 2004 Multiple myeloma. Lancet 363:875–887

Ovarian cancer
Downward J 2004 RNA interference: science, medicine and the future. British Medical Journal 328:1245–1248
McGuire WP, Markman M 2003 Primary ovarian cancer chemotherapy: current standards of care. British Journal of Cancer 89(Suppl 3):S3–S8

Renal cell cancer
Rini BI, Small EJ 2005 Biology and clinical development of vascular endothelial growth factor-targeted therapy in renal cell carcinoma. Journal of Clinical Oncology 23(5):1028–1043

CHAPTER 7

Risk management in drug prescribing

The role of the UK National Patient Safety Agency in improving patient safety is to change practice and systems to reduce risk. It collates data from various organisations and groups across the NHS and issues guidance and advice on how best to deal with errors. Medication errors can be divided into three areas (Avery 2003). Hazardous prescribing, inadequate monitoring and issues at the primary/secondary care interface are common reasons for complications in the prescribing of drugs. Maxwell et al (2002) have listed other more general reasons as to why drug errors may occur, all of which are relevant to the prescribing of anticancer drugs:

- more rapid throughput of patients
- new drug developments, extending medicines into new areas
- increasing complexity of medical care
- increased specialisation
- increased use of medicines generally
- sicker and older patients, more vulnerable to adverse effects.

What is relevant to the prescribing of oral anticancer drugs is that lack of knowledge about a drug and its potential toxicity profiles could easily lead to errors in prescribing. Systems that need to be in place to minimise this risk include good computerised prescribing systems that warn practitioners (e.g. of severe drug interactions) when they prescribe a new drug, and a sound repeat-prescribing policy.

Inadequate monitoring can occur if a patient is not reviewed at the time of a repeat prescription request and systems need to be in place to ensure that repeat prescribing of anticancer drugs is done by expert staff who have the necessary skills and training. Issues around primary and secondary care prescribing usually involve communication breakdown: drug discharge letters that follow a patient after his or her discharge from hospital are often delayed. Secondary care requests by letter for the prescribing of a new drug should be acceptable only if the prescribing doctor is confident about the rationale for the use of the drug, is aware of the potential clinical implications of prescribing and has full knowledge about the monitoring requirements. Similarly, community pharmacists need to be vigilant and check drug dosing and potential interactions that might lead to severe complications. Drug information sheets given out by secondary care to the GP and community pharmacist are a possible method of avoiding significant events. The community pharmacist and GP should accept the need to report near misses as part of the wider reporting culture of monitoring significant events. Errors by community pharmacists have been well documented, including wrong strength of tablets, wrong labelling, the wrong patient receiving the medication and wrong quantities of drug being given.

DRUG INTERACTIONS WITH ANTICANCER DRUGS (*BRITISH NATIONAL FORMULARY LISTED*)

Drug interactions in patients with cancer may be missed if there is lack of knowledge about the potential side effect profiles of anticancer agents. The *British National Formulary* (March 2004) divides drug interactions into pharmacodynamic and pharmacokinetic effects:

- Pharmacodynamic interactions occur between drugs with similar side effect profiles.
- Pharmacokinetic interactions refer to the alteration of the absorption, distribution, metabolism or excretion of the drug by another drug.

The effect of a pharmacokinetic interaction may be to potentiate the action of the drug or reduce its efficacy. Those with reduced renal excretion, the elderly and patients taking drugs with narrow therapeutic windows, such as phenytoin, are those most susceptible to drug interaction. Patients, particularly as inpatients, quite commonly suffer from drug interactions, mainly because they tend to be on a large number of drugs (Riechelman 2004).

Common interactions with anticancer drugs are listed in Table 7.1.

TABLE 7.1 Interactions with anticancer drugs

Drug	Interacting drug	Effect
Antihypertensive drug	Aldesleukin Corticosteroids NSAIDs	Increased hypotensive effects May decrease the antitumour effect Capillary leak syndrome
Alemtuzumab		None known
Aminoglutethimide	Digoxin Dexamethasone Warfarin Phenytoin and phenobarbital	Reduced efficacy of digoxin Increased metabolism of dexamethasone and so reduced effect Reduced anticoagulant effect Increased metabolism of antiepileptic and so reduced efficacy
Anastrozole		No significant interactions
Asparaginase	Methotrexate Vincristine	Reduced action of methotrexate Vincristine-induced neurotoxicity
Azathioprine	ACE inhibitors and angiotensin II antagonists and aminosalicylates Allopurinol Antibacterials, e.g. co-trimoxazole and trimethoprim Anticoagulants	Increased risk of leucopenia Enhanced cytotoxic effect Haematological toxicity Increased anticoagulant effect
Bacille Calmette–Guérin (BCG)	Myelosuppressives Quinolones	Reduced efficacy of BCG Reduced effect of BCG
Carboplatin	Myelosuppressives Aminoglycosides Paclitaxel Amifostine	Increased bone marrow toxicity Increased chance of nephrotoxicity Delayed excretion of paclitaxel if given before paclitaxel Reduced renal clearance of carboplatin
Cisplatin	Amifostine Cytotoxics, e.g. methotrexate Nephrotoxics, e.g. aminoglycosides Paclitaxel	Reduced renal toxicity with cisplatin by inactivation Reduced renal excretion of other cytotoxic agents with associated toxicity Increased renal toxicity Delayed excretion of paclitaxel if given before paclitaxel
Cyclophosphamide	Anticoagulants Anticonvulsants Digoxin Doxorubicin	Enhanced anticoagulant effect Toxic metabolites of cyclophosphamide produced Increased metabolism of digoxin and so reduced effect Increased risk of cardiotoxicity

Continued on page 178

TABLE 7.1 Interactions with anticancer drugs *continued*

Drug	Interacting drug	Effect
Bicalutamide	Anticoagulants	Enhanced anticoagulant effect, needs monitoring
	Antihistamines	Enhanced cytotoxicity
Bleomycin	Cisplatin	Reduced clearance of bleomycin
	Phenothiazines	Reduces activity of bleomycin
	Oxygen	High concentrations of oxygen lead to increased toxicity with bleomycin
Busulfan	Paracetamol	Increased toxicity
	Phenytoin	Metabolism of busulphan increased
Carmustine	Amphotericin B	Increased renal toxicity
	Cimetidine	Side effects of carmustine therapy increased
	Digoxin	Reduced digoxin levels
	Phenytoin	Reduced levels of anticonvulsant
Cytarabine	Alkylating agents	Increased cytotoxicity of alkylating agents
	Digoxin	Reduced plasma levels of digoxin
	Flucytosine	Reduced plasma concentration of flucytosine
	Fludarabine	Raised intracellular concentration of cytarabine
Dacarbazine	Anticonvulsants	Induce microsomal P450 enzymes to reduce effect of dacarbazine
Darbepoetin α	None known	
Daunorubicin	Dexrazoxane	Reduced cardiotoxicity
Daunorubicin (liposomal)	None known	
Dactinomycin-D	None known	
Docetaxel	Antibacterials, antifungals, antihistamines, ciclosporin	Affects the liver P450 system to cause toxicity
Doxorubicin	Antivirals	Inhibition effect of stavudine
	Ciclosporin	Neurotoxicity
Doxorubicin (liposomal)	Anticonvulsants	E.g. phenytoin can increase toxicity
	Cyclophosphamide	Increased risk of cystitis
	Digoxin	Reduced effect of digoxin
Epirubicin	Cimetidine	Cimetidine reduced plasma levels of epirubicin
	Cytotoxics	Increased myelosuppression
Etoposide	Anticoagulants	Enhanced anticoagulant effect
Etoposide phosphate	Anticoagulants	Enhanced anticoagulant effect

TABLE 7.1 Interactions with anticancer drugs *continued*

Drug	Interacting drug	Effect
Exemestane	No drug interactions known	
Filgrastim	Fluorouracil	Increased neutropenia
Fluorouracil	Allopurinol Metronidazole	Avoid Increased toxicity due to increased metabolism
Flutamide	Warfarin	Increased anticoagulant effect
Fludarabine	Cytarabine and other cytotoxics Pentostatin	Effect of these drugs may be enhanced Pulmonary toxicity
Gemcitabine	Cisplatin	Cisplatin toxicity increased
Goserelin	No known interactions	
Hydroxyurea	5-FU Antiretroviral agents	Toxicity with these drugs increased
Idarubicin	Probenecid	Nephropathy
Ifosfamide	Allopurinol Anticonvulsants Warfarin	Toxic metabolites formed Stimulated P450 system leads to increased toxicity with ifosfamide Increased anticoagulant effect
Imatinib	Paracetamol Warfarin Phenytoin, St John's wort Erythromycin, ketoconazole Simvastatin	Avoid Enhanced anticoagulant effect Reduced plasma concentration of imatinib Increased plasma concentration of imatinib Plasma concentration of imatinib increased
Interferon	Theophylline Live vaccines	Theophylline levels increased Contraindicated for 3 months after completing therapy
Irinotecan	No listed drug interactions	
Leucovorin	Anticonvulsants Fluorouracil Methotrexate	Reduced plasma levels of drugs such as phenytoin Cytotoxic action of 5-FU increased Leucovorin rescues from methotrexate toxicity
Letrozole	No interacting drugs	
Leuprolide	No interacting drugs known	
Lomustine	Cimetidine	Side effects of lomustine increased

Continued on page 180

TABLE 7.1 Interactions with anticancer drugs *continued*

Drug	Interacting drug	Effect
Megestrol acetate	Aminoglutethimide, Antibacterials	Lower plasma levels of megestrol
Melphalan	Cimetidine	Reduced concentration of melphalan
	Ciclosporin	Increased risk of nephrotoxicity
Mercaptopurine	Allopurinol	Increased toxicity of mercaptopurine
	Aminosalicylates	Leucopenia
	Co-trimoxazole and trimethoprim	Increased haematological toxicity
	Anticoagulants	Reduced anticoagulant effect
Mesna	Cyclofosfamide and ifosfamide	Reduces the bladder toxicity associated with these compounds
Methotrexate	Nitrous oxide	Increased antifolate effect
	NSAIDs, aspirin	Reduced renal excretion of methotrexate with risk of toxicity
	Co-trimoxazole and trimethoprim	Increased toxicity with methotrexate
	Phenytoin	As above
	Pyrimethamine (antimalarial)	As above
	Ciclosporin	As above
	Corticosteroids	Increased haematological effects
	Acitretin (retinoid)	Increased plasma concentration of methotrexate
	Omeprazole	Increased toxicity of methotrexate
	Warfarin	Increased anticoagulant effect
Mitomycin-C	None known	
Mitoxantrone	Heparin	Incompatible
Mofetil	Aciclovir	Increased plasma levels
Mycophenolate	Cholestyramine, antacids	Reduced absorption
Oxaliplatin	None known	
Paclitaxel	Rosiglitazone	Metabolism of rosiglitazone reduced
Pentostatin	Fludarabine	Contraindicated, fatal pulmonary toxicity
Platinum compounds	Aminoglycosides	Increased risk of nephrotoxicity and ototoxicity
	Amifostine	Reduced renal toxicity with cisplatin Reduced renal clearance of carboplatin
Procarbazine	Alcohol	Nausea, vomiting, headache
	Tricyclic antidepressants	Severe hypertension
Retinoids	Anticoagulants	Reduced anticoagulant effect
	Antiepileptics	Reduced plasma concentration of carbamazepine

TABLE 7.1 Interactions with anticancer drugs *continued*

Drug	Interacting drug	Effect
Retinoids *continued*	Methotrexate	Increased plasma concentration of methotrexate
	Progestogens	Risk of low contraceptive effect
	Vitamins	Risk of hypervitaminosis A
Raltitrexed	Leucovorin	Reduced antitumour effect
Rituximab	No interactions known	
Streptozocin	Steroids	Hyperglycaemia
	Aminoglycosides	Nephrotoxic
Tamoxifen	Anticoagulants	Increased anticoagulant effect
	Aminogluthemide	Reduced plasma tamoxifen levels
Temozolomide	No significant toxicity	
Thalidomide	Alcohol and sedatives	Increased sedation
Thioguanine	No significant interactions	
Thiotepa	Myelosuppressive drugs	Increased bone marrow toxicity
Topotecan	No significant interacting drugs	
Trastuzumab	Anthracyclines	Cardiotoxicity
Tretinoin	Drugs metabolised by liver P450 system	Reduced levels of drug
Vincristine	Itraconazole	Risk of neurotoxicity
	Nifedipine	Reduced metabolism of vincristine
	Cytotoxics	With platinum agents increased renal toxicity
Vinorelbine	Phenytoin	Reduced plasma levels and hence effect of phenytoin

References

Avery AT 2003 Classifying and identifying errors. Pharmaceutical Journal 271:7256

Maxwell S et al 2002 Using drugs safely. British Medical Journal 324:930–931

Riechelman RP 2004 Abstracts of the 40th Annual Meeting of the American Society of Clinical Oncology. New Orleans, Louisiana, USA, 5–8 June 2004. Journal of Clinical Oncology 22(14 Suppl):1s–1069s

Electronic sources of information

GENERAL SOURCES OF INFORMATION FOR PATIENTS AND HEALTHCARE PROFESSIONALS

www.aacr.org
The website of the American Association for Cancer Research.

www.bacr.org.uk
This website lists the activities of the British Association For Cancer Research (BACR).

www.cancerguide.org/online.html
Recommends a number of websites that might be useful for a general explanation of cancer and cancer treatment.

www.cancer.org/
An American Cancer Society website. There are links for patients as well as professionals. The site includes the treatment of cancer and a list of current clinical trials. There is also a section on an interactive version of the National Comprehensive Cancer Networks on the treatment and supportive guidelines for specific tumour types.

www.cancer.gov/cancertopics
This site is run by the National Cancer Institute (NCI) and is very useful in terms of looking at the current evidence for the treatment of specific cancers. It uses the PDQ® database to search for best evidence. There is a search facility for cancer clinical trials. The library contains plenty of material on the complications of cancer and its treatment and there are PDQ® statements relevant both for patients and healthcare professionals.

www.cancerbacup.org.uk
A comprehensive site that covers cancer types, treatments and is relevant both for patients and health professionals. It has a news update section that is also covered by a telephone helpline service. CancerBACKUP is a UK national charitable organisation.

www.cancerindex.org/
A comprehensive directory-type website with listings on the treatment of cancer, journal links and cancer organisations. This site is relevant to healthcare professionals and researchers, as well as to patients. There is quite a lot on cancer chemotherapy but some details are not quite up to date.

www.cancerlinks.org/
A useful site that lists many websites that are cancer specific.

www.cancerresearchuk.org/
The website for Cancer Research UK, an amalgamation of cancer research organisations throughout the UK. There is information about the structure of Cancer Research UK, patient information and plenty on new research currently being undertaken.

www.cancersource.com/
This site seems to cover cancer from childhood to adults, with a section on complementary therapies. The physician database on chemotherapy drugs is particularly useful.

www.cancerscreening.nhs.uk
This is the NHS cancer screening programme website and has information on breast, cervical, colorectal and prostate cancer in particular.

www.nejm.org
This is the site for the *New England Journal of Medicine* and allows access to abstracts on published papers with a search facility.

www.crusebereavmentcare.org.uk
The website for Cruse, a leading charity in the UK specialising in bereavement.

www.ctu.mrc.ac.uk/Browsecancer.asp
The website of the Medical Research Council (MRC) Clinical Trials Unit. It lists open and closed clinical cancer trials.

www.dipex.org
Contains accounts of patients' personal experiences of health and illness, including cancer.

www.ecog.org/

The Eastern Co-operative Group (ECOG) in the United States has the remit of setting up and coordinating multicentre cancer clinical trials. It is funded by the National Cancer Institute and has institutions affiliated to it from across the United States and Canada. The site gives a good introduction on cancer clinical trials, on active clinical trials and protocols and it has the ECOG performance status and common toxicity criteria on its site.

www.eortc.be/

The website of the European Organisation for Research and Treatment (EORTC). It has information about its current active and archived trials and even a small section on complementary and alternative medicine. There is a good section on RECIST in question-and-answer format. There is a good section on the publications produced by the individual EORTC tumour-specific groups.

www.gig.org.uk

The genetics interest group is a UK national alliance of patient organisations with a support children, families and individuals affected by genetic disorders.

www.gog.org/

The website of the Gynaecologic Oncology Group, which is involved in research, both clinical and non-clinical in gynaecologic malignancies. It has links to information on specific malignancies such as using the PDQ® and CANCERLIT® databases.

www.icr.ac.uk/

The Institute of Cancer Research (UK) provides a project database and annual reports of research activities.

www.jco.org/

This is the *Journal of Clinical Oncology* website. It allows access to abstracts of published papers but requires full subscription for full access.

www.macmillan.org.uk

Macmillan cancer relief provides good information on cancer publications and facts for the patient.

www.mariecurie.org.uk

Marie Curie Cancer Care is a cancer charity that provides practical nursing care at home and specialist multidisciplinary care. It has a site for healthcare professionals to access what is available through PCTs.

www.nci.nih.gov/

The website of the National Cancer Institute. This site is useful for providing lots of information on the management of specific tumours with information on clinical trials and relevant cancer litreature. An excellent website.

http://oncolink.org/

The University of Pennsylvania runs this site. It is a comprehensive site that looks at treatment options in relation to different tumour types. It has a good section on how to deal with cancer and its complications from a patient's perspective. There is a link to the major clinical trials websites that are run through America, including the South West Oncology Group. There are links to peer-reviewed cancer journals through (www.oncolink.org/library)

www.patient.co.uk

This patient-orientated portal provides links to many patient groups and self-help links.

www.royalmarsden.org/

The website of the Royal Marsden Hospital. Plenty of information, including details of clinical research work and services at the Hospital, as well as good links to other cancer-related websites. There is a series of online booklets on cancer treatment for the patient.

www.seer.cancer.gov/statistics

The site for Surveillance Epidemiology and End Results (SEER). It provides an excellent source for cancer statistics and tools to calculate statistical enquiries.

www.thpct.nhs.uk/guidetoprescribing/index.html

This guide illustrates local prescribing policies and advice in primary care and across the primary–secondary care interface. It does not expressly mention cancer at the moment but does have good algorithms that aid clinical decision making in drug prescribing.

www.ukcccr.co.uk/

This is the site for the UK Coordinating Committee on Cancer Research (UKCCCR) National Register of Cancer Trials. It allows a search of randomised controlled trials in cancer. The register is managed by the MRC Clinical Trials Unit.

www.21stcenturyoncology.com/cancer

This site provides patients with information on cancer. It talks about specific tumour types but there is perhaps too much detail to take in for the cancer-affected patient.

www.who.int/cancer/

The site of the World Health Organization (WHO). The section on cancer refers to the strategy WHO is taking in cancer prevention and control.

TUMOUR-SPECIFIC WEBSITES

BREAST CANCER

www.breakthrough.org.uk
Breakthrough Breast Cancer is a charity that supports breast cancer research and promotes breast cancer education and awareness.

www.lymphoedema.org
This site advises patients affected by lymphoedema run through the Lymphoedema Support Network.

HODGKIN'S LYMPHOMA, NON-HODGKIN'S LYMPHOMA AND MYELOMA

www.lrf.org.uk
Leukaemia research has produced a good information site on the presentation, staging and management of patients presenting with these tumours as well as the main myeloblastic syndromes.

www.lymphoma.org.uk
This is a website run by the Lymphoma Association, a patient information resource.

www.myeloma.org.uk
This site run by the Internal Myeloma Foundation UK is a useful site for both patients and healthcare professionals.

KIDNEY CANCER

www.kcuk.org
Kidney Cancer UK organises this patient support group.

OESOPHAGEAL CANCER

www.opa.org.uk
The Oesophageal Patients' Association is a patient support group that helps people who have had this disease.

TESTICULAR AND PROSTATE CANCERS

www.orchid-cancer.org.uk
ORCHID cancer appeal aims to raise funds for research and education.

www.prostatecancersupport.co.uk
The Prostate Cancer Support Association (PSA) is a national organisation of self-help and support groups.

OVARIAN CANCER

www.ovacome.org.uk
OVACOME is a charity to help patients with ovarian cancer and is of use for families and health professionals.

ECOG Common Toxicity Criteria

		0	1	2	3	4
Leucopenia	WBC × 10³	≥4.0	3.0-3.9	2.0-2.9	1.0-1.9	<1.0
	Granulocytes/Bands	≥2.0	1.5-1.9	1.0-1.4	0.5-0.9	<0.5
	Lymphocytes	≥2.0	1.5-1.9	1.0-1.4	0.5-0.9	<0.5
Thrombocyto-penia	Plt × 10³	WNL	75.0-normal	50.0-74.9	25.0-49.9	<25.0
Anaemia	Hgb	WNL	10.0-normal	8.0-10.0	6.5-7.9	<6.5
Haemorrhage (Clinical)	-----	none	mild, no transfusion	gross, 1-2 units transfusion/episode	gross, 3-4 units transfusion/episode	massive, >4 units transfusion/episode
*Infection	-----	none	mild, no active Rx	Moderate, localized infection requires active Rx	severe, systemic infection requires active Rx, specify site	life-threatening, sepsis, specify site
Fever in absence of infection	-----	none	37.1°-38.0° C 98.7°-100.4° F	38.1°-40.0° C 100.5°-104.0° F	>40.0° C (>104.0° F) for less than 24 hrs	>40.0° C (>104.0° F) for >24 hrs or fever with hypotension

• Fever felt to be caused by drug allergy should be coded as allergy.
• Fever due to infection is coded under infection only.

		0	1	2	3	4
GU	Creatinine	WNL	<1.5 × N	>1.5-3.0 × N	3.1-6.0 × N	>6.0 × N
	Proteinuria	No change	1+ or <0.3 g% or <3 g/l	2-3+ or 0.3-1.0 g% or 3-10 g/l	4+ or >1.0 g% or 10 g/l	nephrotic syndrome
	Haematuria	neg	micro only	gross, no clots	gross + clots	requires transfusion
	*BUN	<1.5 × N	1.5-2.5 × N	2.6-5 × N	5.1-10 × N	>10 × N

• Urinary tract infection should be coded under infection, not GU.
• Haematuria resulting from thrombocytopenia should be coded under haemorrhage, not GU.

		0	1	2	3	4
GI	Nausea	none	able to eat reasonable intake	intake significantly decreased but can eat	no significant intake	------

		0	1	2	3	4
GI continued	Vomiting	none	1 episode in 24 hrs	2–5 episodes in 24 hrs	6–10 episodes in 24 hrs	>10 episodes in 24 hrs or requiring parenteral support
	Diarrhoea	none	increase of 2–3 stools/day over pre-RX	increase of 4–6 stools/day, or nocturnal stools, or moderate cramping	increase of 7–9 stools/day, or incontinence, or severe cramping	increase of ≥10 stools/day or grossly bloody diarrhoea, or need for parenteral support
	Stomatitis	none	painless ulcers, erythema, or mild soreness	painful erythema, oedema, or ulcers, but can eat	painful erythema, oedema or ulcers, and cannot eat	requires parenteral or enteral support
Liver	Bilirubin	WNL	-----	$<1.5 \times N$	<1.5–$3.0 \times N$	$>3.0 \times N$
	Transaminase (SGOT, SGPT)	WNL	$<2.5 \times N$	2.6–$5.0 \times N$	5.1–$20.0 \times N$	$>20.0 \times N$
	Alk Phos or 5'nucleotidase	WNL	$<2.5 \times N$	2.6–$5.0 \times N$	5.1–$20.0 \times N$	$>20.0 \times N$
	Liver – clinical	no change from baseline	-----	-----	precoma	hepatic coma
	• Viral hepatitis should be coded as infection rather than liver toxicity.					
Pulmonary	-----	none or no change	asymptomatic, with abnormality in PFTs	dyspnoea on significant exertion	dyspnoea at normal level of activity	dyspnoea at rest
	• Pneumonia is considered infection and not graded as pulmonary toxicity unless felt to be resultant from pulmonary changes directly induced by treatment.					

		0	1	2	3	4
Cardiac	Cardiac dysrhythmias	none	asymptomatic, transient, requiring no therapy	recurrent or persistent, no therapy required	requires treatment	requires monitoring, or hypotension or ventricular tachycardia or fibrillation
	Cardiac function	none	asymptomatic, decline of resting ejection fraction by less than 20% of baseline value	asymptomatic, decline of resting ejection fraction by more than 20% of baseline value	mild CHF, responsive to therapy	severe or refractory CHF
	Cardiac – ischaemia	none	non-specific T-wave flattening	asymptomatic, ST and T wave changes suggesting ischaemia	angina without evidence for infarction	acute myocardial infarction
	Cardiac – pericardial	none	asymptomatic effusion, no intervention required	pericarditis (rub, chest pain, ECG changes)	asymptomatic effusion; drainage required	tamponade, drainage urgently required
Blood pressure	Hypertension	none or no change	asymptomatic, transient increase by >20 mm Hg (D) or to >150/100 if previously WNL. No treatment required	recurrent or persistent increase by >20 mm Hg (D) or >150/100 if previously WNL. No treatment required	requires therapy	hypertensive crisis
	Hypotension	none or no change	changes requiring no therapy (including transient orthostatic hypotension)	requires fluid replacement or other therapy but not hospitalisation	requires therapy and hospitalisation, resolves within 48 hours of stopping the agent	requires therapy and hospitalisation for >48 hours after stopping the agent
Skin	-----	none or no change	scattered macular or popular eruption or erythema that is asymptomatic	scattered macular or papular eruption or erythema with pruritus or other associated symptoms	generalised symptomatic macular, papular or vesicular eruption	exfoliative dermatitis or ulcerating dermatitis

	0	1	2	3	4
Allergy	-----	transient rash, drug fever <38° C,100.4° F	urticaria, drug fever ≥38° C, 100.4° F, mild bronchospasm	serum sickness, bronchospasm, requires parenteral meds	anaphylaxis
*Phlebitis		none	arm	thrombophlebitis, leg	hospitalisation	embolus
Local		none	pain	pain and swelling, with inflammation or phlebitis	ulceration	plastic surgery indicated
Alopecia	-----	no loss	mild hair loss	pronounced or total hair loss	----- -	-----
Weight loss	-----	<5.0%	5.0–9.9%	10.0–19.9%	≥20%	-----
Sensory	neurosensory	none or no change	mild paraesthesia, loss of deep tendon reflexes	mild or moderate objective sensory loss; moderate paraesthesia	severe objective sensory loss or paraesthesia that interfere with function	-----
	neurovision	none or no change	----- -	-----	symptomatic subtotal loss of vision	blindness
	neurohearing	none or no change	asymptomatic, hearing loss on audiometry only	tinnitus	hearing loss interfering with function but correctable with hearing aid	deafness, not correctable
Motor	neuromotor	none or no change	subjective weakness, no objective findings	mild objective weakness without significant impairment of function	objective weakness with impairment of function	paralysis
	neuroconstipation	none or no change	mild	moderate	severe	ileus >96 hours
Psych	neuromood	no change	mild anxiety or depression	moderate anxiety or depression	severe anxiety or depression	suicidal ideation

* denotes ECOG specific criteria

		0	1	2	3	4
Clinical	neurocortical	none	mild somnolence or agitation	moderate somnolence or agitation	severe somnolence, agitation, confusion, disorientation or hallucinations	coma, seizures, toxic psychosis
	neurocerebellar	none	slight incoordination, dysdiadochokinesis	intention tremor, slurred speech, nystagmus	locomotor ataxia	cerebellar necrosis
	neuroheadache	none	mild	moderate or severe transient	unrelenting and severe	-----
Metabolic	Hyperglycemia	<116	116–160	161–250	251–500	>500 or ketoacidosis
	Hypoglycemia	>64	55–64	40–54	30–39	<30
	Amylase	WNL	<1.5 × N	1.5–2.0 × N	2.1–5.0 × N	>5.1 × N
	Hypercalcemia	<10.6	10.6–11.5	11.6–12.5	12.6–13.5	≥13.5
	Hypocalcemia	>8.4	8.4–7.8	7.7–7.0	6.9–6.1	≤6.0
	Hypomagnesaemia	>1.4	1.4–1.2	1.1–0.9	0.8– 0.6	≤0.5
Coagulation	Fibrinogen	WNL	0.99–0.75 × N	0.74–0.50 × N	0.49–0.25 × N	≤0.24 × N
	Prothrombin time	WNL	1.01–1.25 × N	1.26–1.50 × N	1.51–2.00 × N	>2.00 × N
	Partial thromboplastin time	WNL	1.01–1.66 × N	1.67–2.33 × N	2.34–3.00 × N	>3.00 × N

Index

Page numbers in *italics* refer to tables; *a* = appendix; *fr* = further reading; *r* = references.